I
KABBALAH

This stimulating approach
the leading authorities on h..
ings of the Kabbalah and visualization in a uniquely ...
form . . .
> **Perle Besserman**, Author of *A New Kabbalah for Women*

Jerry Epstein is a spiritual visionary who has managed to successfully bridge the worlds of tradition and modernity. His work illumines the great Western mystical traditions for contemporary practitioners and explorers. Above all, he includes workable practices so one can move from the intellectual to the experiential dimensions of the tradition, a major contribution toward awakening in our time.
> **E.H. Rick Jarow**, Professor of Religious Studies, Vassar College. Author of *Alchemy of Abundance, Creating the Work You Love*

Dr. Epstein offers an original and insightful work in *Kabbalah for Inner Peace*. He presents in a concise and extremely coherent way what amounts to a new synthesis of Practical and Esoteric Kabbalistic thought: We transcend words (a goal of Esoteric Kabbalah) and turn to self-generated images to effect the physical and spiritual healing as well as improvement of the self (an aspect of Practical Kabbalah). *Kabbalah for Inner Peace* presents a means for connecting to the Divine Other by re-connecting to the innermost self.
> **Ori Z. Soltes**, Professorial Lecturer in Theology and History, Georgetown University. Author of *Our Sacred Signs: How Jewish, Christian and Muslim Art Draw from the Same Source*

This remarkable text is an amazing mental imagery trek from the fragmentation of our lives to connecting upward to the plateaus of the life-giving invisible universe – the universe of visionary, virtual spirituality. The introduction alone is worth the effort – but what follows is life-changing.
> **Ingo Swann**, Renowned Paranormal Researcher. Author of *Natural ESP* and *The Nostradamus Factor*

Dr. Epstein offers readers tantalizing insights into the way Kabbalists have thought about and dealt with the daily worries and pains that beset us. He eloquently describes the tools we need to return to our senses and to root ourselves in our Present. With generosity, he shares short visualizations drawn from his patients' creative responses to restoring balance, patience and freshness to their day. If you wish to lift yourself out of your daily doldrums, do yourself a favor and read this book.

Catherine Shainberg, Ph. D., Author of *Kabbalah and the Power of Dreaming*

Also by Gerald Epstein, M.D.

Healing Visualizations: Creating Health through Imagery

Healing into Imortality: A New Spiritual Medicine of Healing
Stories and Imagery

Climbing Jacob's Ladder: Finding Spiritual Freedom through the
Stories of the Bible

Studies in Non-Deterministic Psychology

Waking Dream Therapy: Unlocking the Secrets of Self through
Dreams and Imagination

Natural Laws of Self-Healing: Harnessing Your Inner Imaging
Power to Restore Health And Reach Spirit (audio)

The Phoenix Process: One Minute a Day to Longevity,
Health & Well-Being (audio)

Other Books by ACMI Press

Alone With The One *by* Colette Aboulker-Muscat
Mea Culpa: Tales of Resurrection *by* Colette Aboulker-Muscat

To my beloved son, Max,
who helped craft the title of the book

KABBALAH FOR INNER PEACE:
Imagery and Insights to Guide You Through Your Day

Gerald Epstein, M.D.

ACMI PRESS : NEW YORK

This book is not intended as a substitute for medical advice of physicians. The reader can consult a physician in matters relating to his or her health and particularly in respect to any symptoms that may require diagnosis or medical attention.

LIBRARY OF CONGRESS CATALOGING-IN-PUBLICATION DATA
Epstein, Gerald, 1935-
    Kabbalah for Inner Peace : Imagery and Insights
    to Guide You Through Your Day / Gerald Epstein.
    p. cm.
    LCCN 2007907049
    ISBN-13: 978-1-883148-08-9
    ISBN-10: 1-883148-08-1

    1. Cabala--Health aspects. 2. Imagery (Psychology)--Therapeutic use. 3. Mind and body.   I. Title.

RZ999.E67 2008   615.8'52
                                 QBI07-600260

Printed in USA.
First Edition
ACMI Press, 2008
351 East 84th Street, #10D
New York, New York 10028
Tel: (212) 369-4080
www.acmipress.org

ACKNOWLEDGMENTS

I wish to thank the wonderful individuals whose support and talent contributed to the writing of this book:

First and foremost, I am indebted to my long-time editor and friend, Harris Dienstfrey. His ability to transform complex ideas into digestible, flowing prose is remarkable. Without him, this book would not be.

I am deeply grateful to Andrea Diamond for her skill and speed in typing, editing, proofreading and preparing the manuscript for final production.

Rachel Epstein, my wife, for her attention to all the details in bringing this project to completion.

Phyllis Kahaney and Sheryl Rosenberg for their comments and revisions.

Al Zuckerman, a literary agent, who encouraged me to pusue the theme of this book.

And, as always, Colette Aboulker-Muscat, my teacher of blessed memory, who initiated me into the path of Visionary Kabbalah, nineteen of whose imagery exercises I have included in this book.

Table of Contents

Introduction.

PRACTICING MENTAL IMAGERY IS PRACTICING KABBALAH

The Relationship Between Spirit and the Everyday World

There are two major ways of understanding the relation between Spirit and the everyday world. In one approach, you find Spirit by drawing away from the everyday world. This is the approach of the East, and it is the approach that many popular books offer to those yearning to bring more spirituality into their lives. While these books don't say that you needn't worry about the chores, tasks and challenges of everyday life, they pay little attention to everyday matters. In these books, what is central is adopting the attitudes and perspectives that take you closer to Spirit by focusing your mind quietly away from the travails of everyday life.

The other approach to the relation between Spirit and daily life is that you move toward the spiritual by bringing it into the everyday. In this approach, mundane life is not a hindrance to Spirit; it is the path to Spirit. You do not turn your back on the chores, tasks and challenges of the everyday, but rather use them to open yourself to Spirit. This is the approach of the West – the approach of "reaching for heaven on earth" – and it is the approach in particular of the path I follow, the path of Visionary Kabbalah. Visionary Kabbalah tells us that to move toward the transcendent we must first gain mastery over our everyday concerns and difficulties.

It is here that we begin to see the conection between inner peace and Spirit. To gain mastery of ourselves in daily life with its bottomless well of challenges requires that we establish in ourselves the inner peace that comes from *balance* and *order*. In this way, gaining inner peace prepares us to open to Spirit. At the same time, the practice of Spirit cultivates inner peace.

The beauty of Visionary Kabbalah is that it offers us several easily available practices that do both – help bring us to inner peace and, at the same time, to the experience of Spirit. Its central practice is mental imagery. Through mental imagery, we enter the realm of the timeless, spaceless Divine, a realm that is always present and available to us, if we only ask. This realm, called the invisible universe, consists of many worlds of reality and beings, e.g., angels, archangels, cherubim.

In this book, I move through typical events and common challenges of an ordinary day and show how mental imagery can help us master our concerns by drawing on Spirit, the source and the essence of our being. In this way we gain inner peace. Not only do we live healthier, calmer, more assured, and more moral lives; but we also put ourselves on the path that leads to transcendence.

I should explain that the Kabbalah I practice is not the Kabbalah that has become a kind of pop hit of the moment, whose study and practice has gained many adherents, a number of them well-known celebrities. This variant is called Ecstatic Kabbalah. About two thousand years old, Ecstatic Kabbalah is based on chanting combinations of Hebrew letters during a meditational state with the aim of bringing the chanter to the transcendent experience of reach-

ing out and up toward union with God. In this
union, one *escapes* the bondage of conditioning and
the enslavement it brings in the time-space physical
reality that we usually, mistakenly, think of as the
only real world. In other words, in this approach to
Kabbalah, one strives to leave behind the ordinari-
ness of human life and leap into the transcendent.

In contrast, Visionary Kabbalah is four to five
thousand years old and derives from the ancient
Western spiritual tradition of the prophets. These
Biblical seers from Abraham onwards describe the
revelatory experiences which came to them in their
visionary practice. In this practice, visions of the
Divine and the transcendent are transmitted via the
sacred language of image. Put another way, image –
and imagery – is the language of the Divine. God
speaks to us through image, and we can reach God
through image. It is a mutual process.

While Visionary Kabbalah is the language of the
Divine it does not mean that the language of image
moves us directly into transcendence. Quite the
contrary. In Visionary Kabbalah, we cannot move
into transcendence until we balance our lives on
earth. Thus, in Visionary Kabbalah, we use image, an
inner hieroglyph, to make God's presence immanent
on earth. We use image to draw on the knowledge
we need to live a healthy, happy, and balanced life.
By applying the revelations that come through
imagery, we transform both our personal lives and
the world around us. Once our inner balance is
secured, we can proceed up the ladder of self-mastery
to make our way first to personal illumination and
then to union with the Divine.

14

Why do I say that image is the sacred language of the Divine?

In Genesis (1:26) it is stated that we are made in the *image* of God. Image in this context represents the indestructible immortal seed we are as created by God. Thus, we bear a cosmic imprint and are open to receiving a continuous influx of Divine energy, which includes information, messages, and light. These influxes come from the invisible world, which is the true reality. Those of us who practice Visionary Kabbalah know it is a science of *revelation* – revelation that is designed to give us peace, comfort, health, and general well-being, from the simplest aspects of our lives to the most complex.
To make God immanent on earth is to bring to earth a new therapeutic impulse that allows us to create a new life, free of conditioning. By transforming our conditioned servitude into freedom, we transform the suffering that usually characterizes daily existence into a life of healing and wholeness.

We can see this process of transformation in the familiar story of Abraham and his encounter with God, about 4,200 years ago in a part of the world that had many tribes, all practicing polytheism – the worship of many gods. People sacrificed fellow humans to propitiate one or another god for whatever benefits the god presumably controlled – rain, crops, cattle, and so forth.

Abraham's encounter with God consisted of his perceiving a great invisible being who in effect said: "I will give you everything that you need on this earth to sustain, fortify, and satisfy you, including eternal health and well-being. All I need in return is your love and devotion."

Mental imagery is akin to Abraham's revelatory experience, which became the basis for the monotheistic tradition.   Imagery puts us in touch with the invisible and thus, according to Abraham's revelation, with what we need in everyday life. Through mental imagery, we access the inner knowledge that helps us heal and brings us back into wholeness; we *remember ourselves* in a new way, bringing ourselves back to life from the suffering that is wearing us down.

Remembering Ourselves Into Wholeness

What does remember ourselves mean? It essentially means coming back to life – *re-membering*. We see this in the vivid story from ancient Egypt, where Isis, the goddess of wisdom, re-members her husband, Osiris. As the god of the netherworld, Osiris weighed the souls of the dead to determine where each soul would go. Osiris's brother, Seth, was so jealous of Osiris's power that he murdered his brother and then cut him into fourteen pieces, burying them all over Egypt.   When Isis learned of this, she scoured Egypt to find the pieces, and after collecting them, she put together all but one of them, restoring Osiris to life.[1] She *re-membered* him. She put his members back together, a process of cosmic reconstructive surgery. Because she recalled him whole, through an act of remembering, *both physical and mental*, she brought him back to life.

---

[1] In the Western spiritual tradition, the woman holds the key to love, which the man learns through her, and so becomes complete.

In mental imagery we re-member and restore ourselves from the fragmentation we experience both internally and externally from the disturbing situations that surround us. We bring ourselves back to life by aligning ourselves with the truths that come to us from the invisible universe. This sacred realm knows what we need and is always available to us through mental imagery.

The revelatory way of the prophets, the systematizers of Visionary Kabbalah, is alive today in the use of mental imagery for purposes of both healing and spiritual realization. This book endeavors to show readers how to invigorate their lives in the spirit of Visionary Kabbalah. In a modest way, the book aims to give everyone the means to become a practicing kabbalist.

A Personal Note

In 1989, I published a book on mental imagery, *Healing Visualizations: Creating Health Through Imagery* (which, I am happy to say, is still in print), without a single word about Kabbalah. Many books on mental imagery take no notice of Kabbalah because the authors either have no spiritual interests or are unaware of the unique connection between imagery and Kabbalah. In my case, I did not discuss Kabbalah because I thought then that placing imagery in what to me was its true and deepest context would ask too much of readers. Healing Visualizations is very much a nuts-and-bolts handbook of imagery treatments for various disorders from acne to worry. In 1989, it seemed enough to me (and my editors) to maintain that imagery could alleviate physical, mental, and emotional disorders.

The world has changed. The use of imagery has gained increasing acceptance. Discussion of the spiritual realities behind the physical realities that come to us through our senses has gained a wide audience – even making some inroads in the medical community, which has begun to study the possible effects of spirituality or belief in God on health. In *Healing Visualizations*, I told only one piece of the story of mental imagery – the story of application. In *Kabbalah for Inner Peace*, I am telling the whole story – that mental imagery is the way that we can access the invisible reality; that our first aim in asking for assistance from this invisible world is to bring balance to our human lives, physically, emotionally and mentally; and that when we do this, in effect, we make God immanent on earth. We have then prepared ourselves to reach out to the transcendent.

Imagery As Prayer

All spiritual tradition speaks about two worlds: the realm of visible reality and the unseen invisible realm. The world of visible reality is the world of time, space, and physicality: that which can be measured and objectified. It is the world of material reality.

The invisible world is a different order of reality operating under different rules. It is the non-space, non-time, pandimensional or multidimensional world.

In the Western spiritual tradition, when we speak of Spirit we refer to the presence, the influence, and the priority of invisibility in our visible world of objective material reality. In this tradition, every image experience is a prayer sent up to invisible reality. Practitioners of Visionary Kabbalah understand that we actively participate in our own physical and spiritual well-being when we engage in our image-prayers. Prayer is not a casual process – "God, let me win the lottery!" It is an act that involves judgment, discernment, decision, and clarity – the four meanings of the Hebrew word for prayer – *tefila*.

But these image-prayers are not always fulfilled in ways we desire. We cannot control the world and its outcomes. We certainly cannot control the invisible reality. But we can take charge of our intentions. And so, we set forth our intentions – we aim toward something desired via image-prayer. Yet even as we do this, we recognize that the outcome, result, goal, or endpoint is in God's hands, not our own. From the perspective of Visionary Kabbalah, whether or not an image-prayer is fulfilled, the invisible universe provides us what we need at every given moment.

When we are aligned with truth and have faith in the invisible reality, we receive what we need in the form of support. When we have no faith and veer from the truth, we receive what we need in the form of experiences like pain or other imbalances that show us the error of our ways and give us the opportunity to correct them.

The Four Planes of Existence: Vertical Causality

In Visionary Kabbalah, the physical reality of the world and our bodies is, in a manner of speaking, at the bottom of the totem pole of creation. Causality, in the perspective of Kabbalah, goes from top down – not as we commonly think of it and as the natural sciences of the physical world say it operates – from bottom up.

ALL INFINITE BEING = THAT WITHOUT END = GOD

INVISIBLE

IMPULSE — EMANATION

IDEA — CREATION

IMAGE — FORMATION

VISIBLE

Physical World/body ← ACTION → Experience Emotions

VERTICAL CAUSALITY

HORIZONTAL CAUSALITY
Physical Time and Space

There are four planes of existence in Kabbalistic cosmology, each giving birth to (causing) the plane below it. This is called vertical causality, and all four planes operate in both the cosmos and our individual lives. Cosmologically, the top plane is what Visionary Kabbalah calls *emanation* or invisible reality, which gives birth to (causes) *creation*, which gives birth to (causes) *formation*, which gives birth to (causes) *action* – the realm of the physical world and the physical body. Each of these four planes is reflected in our individual lives. *Emanation* in our lives is the realm of the will, or spark of life. *Creation* is the realm of ideas, beliefs and concepts. *Formation* is the realm of image. *Action* is the realm of experience and emotion. Just as *emanation* (invisible reality) leads to *creation*, which leads to *formation*, which leads to the physical world – in effect, to us; will, the spark of life, leads to ideas, which leads to image, which leads to experience and emotion. The same vertical causality that operates in the cosmos operates in us as well. As the invisible reality creates the visible world, we create our experience.

All this is illustrated in the preceding chart.

In the physical world in which we live, experience has the qualities of volume, mass and duration, which means that it is susceptible to being measured, calculated, or otherwise quantified. Experience gives us an opportunity to know what is going on inside of us. At the same time, it can be actively and consciously created by us, from inner to outer, through a working or re-working of our inner concepts and images. As we have seen, *formation* gives birth to *action* in the physical world. In this world as we live it, our images give birth to our experience. Thus, by changing our inner concepts and images, we influence, shape, or reshape our outer reality. The beauty of this is that in terms of the creation of physical existence, we are at the bottom of the totem pole, yet we have the tools – our concepts and images – to create and recreate our lives and lift ourselves upward to the world of Spirit. We come from what is higher, and through our images and concepts, we can rise back up to that which is our true being.

A primary symbol of kabbalistic wisdom is the tree. We are to be as a tree in establishing a spiritual direction. A tree must first be planted firmly in the ground and create roots so that it remains firmly planted and not break or become uprooted when beset by the elements. Being firmly rooted, it can grow up to the sky and radiate endlessly upward and outward.

This book's direction

This book starts the process of our becoming as a tree. Using the language of Spirit, we bring the force of Spirit to bear on everyday life. In a phrase, we bring there (Spirit) here (everyday living) to change our ongoing life, which is the ground from which we can make our way up the ladder of self-mastery to reach toward Spirit.

Let me be more matter-of-fact. In Visionary Kabbalah, the body is the temple of the Spirit, the Spirit's house. Without the body, there is no possibility for discovering Spirit. At the same time, we are not to make the body into an idol. What we are to do is take care of it and keep it healthy, so that it serves as a secure base to move toward Spirit.

As we treat our bodies, so we should treat the whole of our lives. We keep ourselves healthy and happy and balanced – a fundamental concept in Visionary Kabbalah – because if we don't, then we damage our chance to move toward the life of Spirit and the reality of the invisible universe. In so doing, we neither idolize our physical lives nor worship Mammon. (The ancients considered Mammon the personification of avarice and worldly gain.) Rather, we show respect to our lives, and fill them with the abundance of well-being in its many forms.

I have arranged the material in this book to mimic the passage of a representative day in which we face the tasks and challenges of ordinary living. I want to show how we can invest our lives at all points with health and happiness, balance and abundance. To this end, there are imagery exercises to start the day and imagery exercises to end it. In between, I cover many common concerns about the material and physical conditions of our lives, our relationships, and our spiritual aspirations: worries about money; everyday ailments such as anxiety, pain, and self-doubt; and interpersonal disturbances with our bosses (who can exert heavy influences over our lives) as well as with some of the people who are dearest to us (spouses, children, parents). Where it is appropriate, I show how to reach outward into the larger reality of Spirit.

Central to all this is the kabbalistic principle illustrated in the chart above – that what we believe is what we manifest as our experience in our earthly time-space dimensional reality. As we have seen, what we conceive in our thoughts and imagination gives birth to our experiential world. Image – the belief/concept given form – is the intermediary and the method of this birthing process. Once the image is perceived in the inner forum of our consciousness, it gives us direction, guidance and new understanding for carrying out our lives.

Image, however, is a double-edged sword. On the one hand, it can bring us health and balance; on the other hand, it can turn us away from Spirit and balance. We usually are unaware of the damaging images that we hold (of our capabilities, for example, or the worth of others). But we can become aware of them, and then, with conscious and deliberate mental imagery, change the damaging images, replacing them with the images that we want to influence our lives. Making such changes is a critical part of our daily lives if we want to move toward balance and Spirit.

In this book, I hope to set out the way in which imagery enables us to call on our true inner power, to clean out the obstacles obstructing our natural flow of harmony, and to put ourselves on the path of self-mastery, freedom and transcendence. The practice of mental imagery is easy to learn and easy to do. We do not need a special place, outwardly or inwardly, or special clothing, or a special ritual. For all practical purposes, imagery can be done anywhere, anyplace, anytime.

The imagery exercises are also very fast. Most take only a matter of seconds, none lasts more than several minutes. This is the homeopathy of the mind in touch with Spirit. Micro amounts of time in the mind engender or stimulate a macro response in both the everyday three-dimensional realm and the spiritual realm from which the everyday arises.

What I offer here has nothing to do with proselytizing or correcting anyone. Rather, it is a way to experiment actively in/with Spirit in an everyday setting. As an active meditation – or a meditation in action – it permits us to take charge of our inner state of being, to gain more understanding of the purpose of living, and to bring abundance into our lives, in ways we may not yet have experienced.

Abundance in this most acquisitive society, I hasten to add, does not mean just material gain and acquisition. Abundance also means becoming happy, peaceful and able to weather the storms of everyday life. We come to "bear the slings and arrows of outrageous fortune" with geniality; able to carry our burdens lightly; to wear our yokes easily, and live a life of law and love within the confines of this lawless and painfully unloving, often heartless world. My hope is that *Kabbalah for Inner Peace*, rooted in the power of Spirit, and the power of image to bring us toward Spirit, sets each of us on the road to fulfilling these possibilities.

Chapter 1.

LEARNING THE PRACTICE OF MENTAL IMAGERY: THE TREATMENT THAT OFTEN TAKES ONLY SECONDS

The Western spiritual tradition, of which Kabbalah is a part, holds that we are born with free will and choice and, at the same time, are participating in a grand cosmic plan that is already blueprinted and is inexorably moving toward its fulfillment. Each of us lives out his or her part of the plan. When we go astray from our inherent divinity, the universe reveals this to us and provides us with the knowledge we need about ourselves.

This knowledge is revealed to us in the language of image. We always experience imaginally every event we encounter, whether the event is external, as in the direct waking experience of the physical world, or internal, as in daydreams, hallucinations, night dreams or imagery experiences that we initiate. It is through such imagery – prayers to the invisible reality – that we can enter the inner life, which holds the cure to our emotional and physical imbalances and the promise of harmony between body, mind, and, eventually, Spirit. It is a central tool by which we seek to better our lives and bring abundance into them.

During the course of this book, we will see people using imagery in their everyday lives for many purposes – to heal physical ailments, to heal the past, to improve relations with other people, to deal with worries and alarms of the present, to assuage long-standing unhappiness, to reach out to Spirit.

Imagery, you might say, is the all-purpose antibiotic of the inner beliefs that direct our passage in the world and shape our physical, social, mental, and moral response to the world.

This is the reason that mental imagery often takes its practitioners far beyond the immediate concern of the moment. People can start with specific problems, but in the course of using imagery to deal with the problem at hand, they may discover the beliefs or situations that limit their reach. This new awareness then provides them with the opportunity to change their beliefs to become who they want to be.

A young freelance graphic artist came to see me because he was having difficulty completing an important assignment that could be a major boost for his career. Although he was a habitual procrastinator, when a deadline loomed, he said, he always had been able to sit himself down and do what needed to be done. This time he couldn't seem to do it. He felt intensely agitated and worried. He desperately did not want to fail. Could I help him?

The Room of Creativity

I suggested an imagery exercise called The Room of Creativity. In this exercise, the young man sees himself entering an elevator that goes down below the earth's surface. He presses the number 5 button. As the elevator descends, he sees the descending numbers light up – 1, 2, 3, 4, 5. At 5, the doors open, and he is in a brightly lit hallway at the end of which is a door. He walks the hallway to the door and sees on the door in gold letters his name: _____'s Room of Creativity. He opens the door, goes inside, and observes the room. He goes to the center, where he finds his graphics table and supplies. He sits there and does his work with facility and ease. After finishing his work, he looks around in order to remember the room. He goes out the door, closes it, and walks the hallway back to the elevator. He gets in and pushes G. The door closes, and he watches the buttons light up as he ascends . . . 5, 4, 3, 2, 1, G. The door opens, and he emerges ready to create in his daily life. He opens his eyes, knowing he has found his special room.

I recommended that he do the exercise once a day in the early morning, with the intention of connecting with his creative energy in graphic design.

We did the exercise once before he left. He said he found it calming.

A week later, he called to tell me that his work was going well. He was feeling confident that he would meet his deadline. He thanked me, even though, he added, he wasn't sure what had happened. Few practices in life are easier than mentally imaging.

How to Start

Mental imagery can be done virtually anywhere, except for those situations in which you need to be alert and need your eyes open for your own safety, e.g. driving a car. Otherwise, more or less anywhere you are – in a subway, on a park bench, in your office, or anywhere you can be sitting up – is an acceptable place to do an imagery exercise. Still, as a rule and especially if you are starting out, it is best to begin your practice in a quiet place, sitting in a chair in a pose that I call the Pharaoh's Posture. (See illustration) *Unless otherwise specified, assume this posture when you are doing imagery. After the first few exercises, I no longer remind you to sit up straight.*

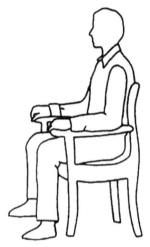

Throughout the ages, the Pharaoh's Posture was assumed by royalty who sought their inner guides before making a decision. It is a posture expressing the search for inner guidance.

You sit straight up in a chair, with your back straight and your feet flat on the floor. Ideally, the chair has arm rests on which you can place your arms; but if you are using a chair without arms, put your hands palms down, flat on your thighs. Do not cross your arms, and do not cross your legs. Make sure your back is straight with your shoulders back.

In the Pharaoh's Posture, you want to blot out the external world. Close your eyes if you are comfortable doing so. Some of you may find that you are not, and if that is the case, keep them open. Closing your eyes removes yourself from external distractions, and permits you to turn inward.

A straight-backed chair is best because a straight spine permits a sense of awareness and alertness to ensue. We become more awake. This posture is the opposite of the horizontal one, which is the habitual one of sleep. Sitting with your back straight also enhances your breathing – your lungs need a vertical posture to expand fully. Awareness of breath, as all ancient physicians and healers knew, promotes greater alertness and attentiveness to mental processes. We become more attuned to our inner life as we become more conscious of our breathing. This is a key to this work.

How to Breathe

We do a special kind of breathing to initiate the process of mental imagery – out-in, not in-out. We breathe *out* long, slow exhalations through the mouth, then breathe *in* brief inhalations through the nose. Long, slow exhalations through the mouth, brief inhalations through the nose.

The long, slow exhalations open the door to the channel that allows the images to emerge in your consciousness. For this reason, concentrate on making your exhalations longer and slower than your inhalations. When you exhale long and slow, it makes you calm and quiet inside. It is the quickest way, in fact, to reduce anxiety; and it is the simplest exercise I know to rid yourself of an anxious state when it arises. Anxiety aside, you need a quiet state of mind in order to focus on the inner work of imagery.

You start with an out breath. You breathe out a long, slow exhalation, and follow it with a brief inhalation. You do this three times – an exhalation followed by an inhalation, an exhalation followed by an inhalation, an exhalation followed by an inhalation. Once you complete this cycle, you need not concentrate on your breathing, and your breathing can assume any pattern that is comfortable for you. During your imagery work, your attention will be focused on the images and your breathing will take care of itself. I stress exhalation over inhalation because breathing to quiet the body begins with an *outbreath*, not an *inbreath*. The more usual in-out breathing stimulates you by exciting the sympathetic or excitatory nervous system and the adrenal medulla, which secretes adrenaline. Out-in breathing, on the other hand, stimulates the parasympathetic nervous system and the vagus nerve, which help the body quiet down.

When an imagery event is over, you take one outbreath before opening your eyes. An outbreath induces an inner quietness. Because we experience some inner stimulation when we engage in an imagery exercise, we want to come back to everyday life in a quiet way. The one outbreath helps take us from an inner focus out to our external life and, by quieting us, gives us a centered place in the physical world. *After the first introductory exercises, I abbreviate the special breathing with the words "breathe out three times slowly" or simply "breathe out."*

How to Begin Imagery

There are three elements to beginning imagery.

First, *you say the name of the exercise to yourself, either inwardly or outwardly* (whichever you find most comfortable). The examples of imagery exercises I provide each have a name. Once you start practicing imagery, you likely will develop your own exercises, and you will see that you more or less naturally give them names.

Second, *you give the exercise an intention.* Throughout the book, I have stated an intention with each exercise. You are always free to modify the intention; whatever your intention, always state it in the present. By intention, I do not mean a goal. Be careful not to confuse an intention with a goal. A goal is always in the future, and Kabbalah tells us that we do not attach ourselves to a goal – that is, act as if we can control our outer life. Intention, on the other hand, is in the here and now. It is concerned with a process, not a product. We want to stay in the present and not burden ourselves with what we cannot know or predict: namely, the future. Our aim is to take charge of our inner life, particularly our beliefs. As I briefly explained in the introduction, a central tenet of Kabbalah is that what we believe will manifest as our experience in the outer world of this time-space dimensional reality. In the next chapter, we look more carefully at the difference between an intention and a goal and how we can have an intention without a goal.

Third, *you set your biological clock by saying (again inwardly or outwardly) how long the exercise is to take.* Our exercises tend to be short, on the order of a few seconds, though some may be longer, occasionally lasting up to a few minutes.

The general rule is: *Do each exercise quickly!* The value of imagery is in the light shock that it gives to your system, which creates a movement we call "life" and promotes healing. You need only a spark. It takes only the flame of one small match to set off all the fireworks. Healing is prompted by this sudden jolt. Healing through imagery is like the homeopathic process in that a minute, micro-amount of substance stimulates the body's macro-healing response.

The rule of thumb for imagery work is that less is more. The shorter the imagery, the stronger its power. The shorter the time in which a given exercise can be done – some imagery exercises necessarily are longer than others – the better. For those of you whose rhythm is naturally longer, give yourself extra seconds, but, <u>not too long.</u> Otherwise, the power of the image can be compro-mised.For long exercises you can make a tape of your voice giving the exercise. After a few times you wont need the tape.

How to Do an Imagery Excercise

Let us put this all together with two imagery exercises. The first deals with physical health – the well-being of our body; the second deals with reach-ing toward the invisible reality – the well-being of turning to Spirit.

I call the first *The Ice Cubes Exercise.* It comes from my book *Healing Visualizations,* and people use it to reduce and control high blood pressure.

The Ice Cubes Exercise

High blood pressure is usually associated with anxiety, anger, and ambition. The process is some-thing like this: As we push ourselves to satisfy our desires, we find ourselves "burning up." In hypertension, our blood and anger are boiling over and have to be cooled down. You will see the relevance of this description in the imagery of the exercise.

You are sitting in a chair in the Pharaoh's Posture. You close your eyes if you feel comfortable doing this. As with each exercise, you breathe out in long, slow exhalations through the mouth and breathe in briefly through the nose, three times. Your intention is that you are doing The Ice Cubes Exercise to reduce your blood pressure and bring it back to normal, and you are doing the exercise up to 15 seconds.

Imagine yourself going to your refrigerator and taking out three or four ice cubes. Wash your head, skull, face, and neck with the ice, and sense and feel the coolness coursing through every pore and entering your bloodstream in the brain. See this ice-blue coolness circulating down from the brain through the neck, down into your trunk, into and through your upper and lower extremities, and out to the tips of your fingers and toes. See and sense the flow of blueness. Know that when you see and sense this ice-blue coolness reaching to your fingertips and toes, your blood pressure has returned to normal.

Now breathe out and open your eyes (if they are closed).

If you have high blood pressure, you may
find that with such a longstanding chronic problem, doing the imagery exercise once is not
enough. With problems that took some time to
develop, we often do an exercise three times a
day for up to 21 days. As a point of kabbalistic
practice, do the exercise at sunup (or when you
arise), sundown, and before going to sleep –
three daily transition points that are considered
natural healing times in many cultures of the
world. We do the exercise for up to or through
21 days because, kabbalistically, the number 21
has the meaning of healing, and you will see
that in many instances, it takes up to three
weeks for a healing to take place.

Of course, it may happen before then. That
is why we say "up to" 21 days. You are giving
yourself up to a three-week period of time for a
healing to happen.

The next series of exercises is called *Self-
Restoration.* Its purpose is to help you make the
turn to the invisible reality, our spiritual source.
The exercise was developed by my teacher,
Colette Aboulker-Muscat, one of the twentieth
century's great healers.

Self-Restoration

Close your eyes and sit in the
Pharaoh's Posture. Breathe out three times
slowly. See, sense, feel and live the well-
known phrase: "Vanity, vanity, all is vanity." Breathe out one time slowly. Become
aware of the vanity in ourselves as the false

picture we are constantly constructing as a way to gain self-fulfillment.

Breathe out one time slowly. Live how self-fulfillment for you usually is asking for immediate or more immediate gratification. Breathe out one time slowly. Live and know how it is a desire to get, and not a desire to give. Breathe out and open your eyes.

Close your eyes. Breathe out one time slowly. Then, see and feel the difference for your self-fulfillment between self-search and self-indulgence. Breathe out and open your eyes.

Close your eyes. Breathe out three times slowly. Live some self-denial as self-gratification. Know now how self-denial does pay off. Breathe out and open your eyes.

Close your eyes. Breathe out three times slowly. Know how the slightest form of pride, as your defense of vanity, is preventing you from seeing the truth. Breathe out one time slowly. Now, as vanity and pride recede, know how humility takes their place. Breathe out and open your eyes.

How You Know Your Imagery Has Had an Effect

There are several ways to know that an imagery exercise has brought about some transformation. You may feel a general sense of lightness. You may have a feeling of renewal and greater energy. Within the imagery process, you may see a golden aura form around you and/or see yourself filling with golden light.

Beyond the immediate moment, you likely will feel changes in the way you live in the world, especially in the confidence you have in yourself. I can report that, generally speaking, imagery is one of the best methods for strengthening our faith and trust in ourselves.

A good example of this is the young woman who came to see me for an infertility problem. Tests had shown that she had normal fallopian tubes, so she could not understand why she so far had been unable to conceive.

I recommended that she do two kinds of imagery exercises, the first with the intention of becoming pregnant, the second with the intention of discovering whether a physical problem was preventing conception. Through the second exercise, she saw that the end of one fallopian tube near the ovary was sealed, crusted over by adhesions and scar tissue, the origin of which she could not explain. Nonetheless, if her imagery was correct, she uncovered a physical-mechanical incapacity of her fallopian tubes. She said nothing to her gynecologist, since she felt he would not believe her, though she did try to clean the crusted-over tube using imagery.

Eventually, she decided to have a fallopian tube transplant in which an egg is fertilized in the tube through a surgical procedure. When her lower abdominal region was opened for this surgery, the tube was found to be in exactly the condition she discovered through her imagery work.

After the operation, the young woman was awed and amazed to find that she knew more about her body (indeed, herself) than did her doctors. She immediately felt increased confidence in her intuition and grew more trusting of her judgment.

I have consistently seen similar beneficial changes in many people who have used imagery to resolve problems and increase their well-being. What is happening here? The power of kabbalistic practice is the immediacy with which we can use imagery to draw on the never-ending sustenance and energy of the invisible reality as the source of our healing of everyday difficulties; simultaneously it enables us to climb the ladder of self-mastery, basic to any effort to rise toward Spirit.

Chapter 2.

THE KABBALAH OF MENTAL IMAGERY:
WORKING WITHOUT A GOAL

In the previous chapter, I explained that when we use imagery, we do it with an intention, but without a goal. This apparent paradox is at the heart of the kabbalistic perspective.

In Kabbalah, an individual gives up his or her quest for achieving an outcome and leaves the outcome to the invisible reality. In the life of Spirit, we are not interested in goals; we are not interested in bringing things to a head or to a conclusion. These functions belong to the domain of God. What we are interested in is opening ourselves to the invisible reality and letting it intervene for us. God said to Abraham and through Abraham to all of us: "I'll give you everything, for the invisible reality is an endless resource. It's limitless, it's infinite, it's eternal. And if you open yourself up to it, it will give you everything, but you have to open yourself up to it. And, remember, I am in charge of goals, results, outcomes." Foregoing goals means accepting the existence – and the abundance – of Spirit.

If we are interested in an outcome, we block the path to healing because we block the invisible world from moving in to help and support us. The invisible world loves us, and it wants to give us everything, but we have to let it operate. If we are goal-oriented, we have co-opted the function of the invisible world; we have usurped the knowledge and power of God.

A woman came to see me because her husband wanted a divorce. He told her he was unhappy. He felt that their daily life lacked "tang." It seemed to him they were living the life of robots. On the other hand, she explained, she was very happy with her married life. She loved routine, orderliness, repetition. That was why she liked chain restaurants, she said: "You always knew what to expect." She couldn't imagine a life filled with impulse. There was a time when her husband would call in the afternoon and suggest they go out for dinner. She never liked that. It unsettled her. She always planned her meals for a full week. To go out basically on a moment's notice would upset her schedule. She liked to go out to restaurants she knew, she said, but she needed to know a week or two ahead of time.

She wanted me to give her an imagery exercise that would make her husband change his mind. She wanted her life to continue as it was. She saw no reason why it could not and should not.

I said that I could not help her. Leaving aside the moral problem of one person controlling another or intruding on or interfering with another's freedom – as she seemed to want to do concerning her husband – I could not in good faith guarantee that in our work she would succeed in fulfilling her absolute commitment to a fixed goal. That fulfillment was between her and the "Creator." In the process I was offering her, we could focus only on her intention, that is, her aim or direction.

The woman was shocked. Several people she knew had recommended me. I had helped them. She didn't understand why I couldn't help her.

I told her I could suggest an imagery exercise that she could practice with the intention of holding her marriage together. The woman said that she did want to hold her marriage together. She also didn't want it to change. I said I could help her with the first desire but not the second.

She sat for a while, then said that if that was all I could provide, she would try the exercise to hold the marriage together. The exercise I gave her follows below.

The Marriage Tree

> Close your eyes. breathe out three times slowly. Know you are doing this exercise with the intention of bringing unity back to your marriage and it is taking 15-20 seconds. See you and your spouse standing on either side of a large tree. See the two of you beginning to grow up alongside the tree, finding yourselves becoming taller than the tree. Then, see, sense, and feel your hearts melding and your arms intertwining. Know that you two are becoming bonded. Breathe out and open your eyes.

I recommended that she do the exercise once a day in the morning for twenty-one days.

The woman did not thank me when she left my office, and I never heard from her again.

While I have no way of knowing the outcome of this rather complex situation, the exercise I offered the woman is a good example of the difference between intention and goal. It also shows that the instruction not to use an intention to achieve a specific goal does not mean that, imaginally speaking, we do nothing and passively wait for something to happen. Kabbalistic practice says that we act and take steps to heal ourselves and then bring that healing impulse to others. We do what we can to bring balance to life.

In this woman's case, I can say she showed no clear sign of wanting to heal herself or bring balance to her life. She wanted the life she wanted, seemingly at whatever cost to herself and others; and she wanted time to stand still. I believe the exercise could have moved her toward healing and a new life for herself, along with a new life for her marriage. But she needed to do the exercise to bring about such movement.

Intention, as I said in the previous chapter, is concerned with "process not product." This is a shorthand way of framing the essence of the spiritual perspective of the kabbalistic system and of what Kabbalah sees as a key to attaining health. Product means the endpoint or goal. Process means focusing on the practice or technique you are doing. Your *intention* is your aim to heal, but your *attention* is on what you are doing to accomplish it. Your task is to focus on the process of taking charge of how you think. You approach the day with the faith that what then comes is what you need: in other words, the universe will support you.

In the kabbalistic perspective, when you practice mental imagery to heal yourself – emotionally, physically, spiritually – you are setting yourself on a *path* of healing. "Path" is the critical word. That is all there is to the practice of mental imagery – a path of healing, not an outcome. If you want to strive for goals or want reassurance that you can control the world around you, from the kabbalistic perspective you probably have the wrong book.

A Zen Exercise of Mental Imagery for Experiencing Process, Not Product

Understanding the important difference between intention and goal is one thing. Practicing it is another. I believe that the following imagery exercise can help you integrate the difference between intention and goal. The exercise has its origins in a book that was a best-seller years ago: Eugene Herrigel's *Zen in the Art of Archery*, which can still be found in many bookstores.

Herrigel explains how a Zen master becomes a qualified and expert archer. The book goes into great detail describing how the Zen master prepares himself to shoot an arrow, how he sets his posture, how he sets his bow, and so on – all of which he does free of any concern with the outcome of his practice. His intention is to shoot the arrow as correctly as he can, and everything he does centers on that intention. As he releases the arrow he *closes* his eyes. After, he opens his eyes to see the arrow has landed in the bull's-eye!

In the next imagery exercise, you do what the Zen master does – shoot the arrow with intention but no goal.

The Zen Master Exercise

Close your eyes and find yourself sitting in the Pharaoh's Posture. Breathe out three times slowly, knowing that you are learning to concentrate on intentions instead of goals and that it takes 30 to 45 seconds.

Now see yourself as your own Zen master. See yourself dressed in a robe with an obi sash tied around it. You have with you a golden bow and a golden quiver that holds one golden arrow. The target is in front of you. You arrange yourself now to shoot the arrow at the target. If you are left-handed, you set your right shoulder perpendicular to the target. If you are right-handed, you set your left shoulder perpendicular to the target.

Your rear foot is pointed in the same direction as you are standing. Your front foot is turned 90 degrees, to face the target. Your posture is quite straight. You sense and feel yourself tall and erect. You are breathing evenly and regularly.

And you now remove the golden arrow from its quiver, which is slung over your shoulder. You take the arrow and you turn your bow in a 45-degree angle upwards and put the golden arrow into the bow. You set the end of the arrow into the string of the bow, hold the wooden frame of the bow very tightly, and pull the string back with your dominant hand, very tautly and tightly, with great strength.

Then, you set the bow at a 90-degree angle facing the target. Still maintaining the same posture, you turn your head to look at the target. You turn right if you are left-handed, you turn left if you are right-handed. You look directly at the bull's eye. Breathe out one time slowly.

You are there in front of the target. You

are about to release the arrow, and just before you do, there in the image, close your eyes so you no longer see the target, and release the arrow. Then breathe out and open your eyes in the image to see where the arrow has landed. See what happens.

Breathe out and open your eyes.

I would think most of you who have done this exercise found that you hit the target. A great many of you may even have hit the bull's-eye. So, you now see and understand that you can achieve what you are aiming for without having to be concerned that you be in control of the result of your effort. By closing your eyes in the image when you release the arrow, you no longer are involved with the outcome of where the arrow goes.

What of those of you who have missed the target altogether? For you, this result is a diagnostic indicator of how much you may be attached to outcomes. If this is the case, I would recommend you do this exercise regularly each morning upon awakening until you finally hit the target – which I believe you ultimately will as you loosen your hold on needing or wanting outcomes.

To those who are fixed on outcomes, a form of dependency which from a kabbalistic perspective is tantamount to enslavement, I would recommend that you practice a variant of this exercise every morning for three weeks. When you take the arrow out of the quiver, write your intention on the shaft of the arrow. And then, after you write it on the shaft, continue the exercise of putting it in the bow, fitting it on the string, and then doing the shooting.

I recommend that you do this exercise every morning before you start your day because it is giving you a new attitude to take with you into the coming day and, so, gives that day a new direction.

You may be very surprised to discover what happens, because soon you are going to see that the universe will enter into your life in a way that you have never experienced before. Things will start coming to you; things that you have been desiring and that have been eluding you will start happening for you. At the same time, you will have a sense of peace, contentment, and fulfillment.

For much the same reason, I would recommend that people who hit the target in their imagery also practice the *Zen Master Exercise* every morning for three weeks. I have seen that most people who start their days with this exercise have found themselves in a new relationship with their everyday life. Within a seven-day period, and almost always within a twenty-one day period, their lives acquired a new abundance.

When we give up our goals and concentrate diligently on the practices of our lives, we increase self-mastery and move toward the invisible universe, toward Spirit, to receive the wonders and miracles the universe has to offer us. This process of *receiving* is exactly what the term Kabbalah means.

Chapter 3.

EXERCISES FOR BRINGING FRESHNESS TO THE DAY

We start our Kabbalah-oriented journey through the day at the obvious place – with rising in the morning.

I cannot emphasize too much that Visionary Kabbalah is always concerned with bringing the healing aid of the invisible reality to bear on our everyday life. A central purpose of Kabbalah is to bring a therapeutic healing to the world – a world that is suffering, in bondage, and subject to brutality day after day.

This healing is ours for the doing. With the tool of mental imagery, each of us can actively set ourselves on the path of vigor and health, every day – from the moment we arise to the moment we lay ourselves down to sleep.

What precisely can we do when we wake to help bring *life* to our lives? Admittedly, relatively few of us are eager to rise. More of us, under the strains of our daily existence, feel that getting up is a burden, something we are not eager to do. Most of us, I suspect, rise, in effect, out of habit. It is something we do because we do it. We do not give it much thought. We enter the day, and then let the day take us over. We let ourselves be carried away on its stream.

You will be interested in the reaction of one person I worked with when he became aware of the extent to which life was leading him. He became so determined to lead himself that he regularly began changing all the morning routines that had marked his waking for years. He saw that he always had shaved with his left hand, always beginning on his left cheek. Now, he alternated hands – at first every other morning, then on a more spontaneous pattern – and kept changing where he began shaving. If he was using his left hand, he started shaving under his chin or under his nose or across his right jaw. When he shaved two or three days in a row using the same hand (so that he wouldn't fall into the pattern of routine alternation), he usually, though not always, followed different shaving patterns.

He applied the same approach to dressing. Instead of always putting his right leg in his pants first, he alternated legs. Sometimes, he even sat on his bed and put both feet in at once. Sometimes he put his socks on before putting on his pants, sometimes after. Sometimes he put on one sock, then put on his pants, then put on the other sock!

You get the picture. He was determined not to be dulled by routine. He insisted on approaching his life actively and deliberately. Eventually, he relaxed this constant application of active consciousness to his morning routines. He saw he did not always need it, that he could fall into routine sometimes without any damage – so long as he took himself out of the routine whenever he wanted to. He saw that as far as preparing himself physically for the day was concerned, he could choose either routine or expanded awareness. It was his choice. And he saw that there were always new places in his life, often more important places, where he could strive to apply awareness to his behavior and his choices.

Still, for the several years that I was in touch with him, he continued the 21-day cycles of beginning his day with an imagery exercise – at first one or another of the exercises I recommended to him, then branching out to exercises of his own making. He wanted to be always ready to put his best foot forward to meet whatever would come to him during the day. He wanted to always respond with vigor and confidence.

Here are two exercises I initially presented to him for this purpose. You can do either exercise. Or, like the man, you can do one on one day, the other the next day, and then maybe do an exercise you devise for yourself on another day. Follow any pattern that suits you. You are your own best guide to the healing therapeutic awareness that helps you become the master of your life and sets you on the path toward Spirit.

As you shall see, both exercises have broader applications than bringing vigor and enthusiasm to your day.

The Question Mark Exercise

Like nearly all mental imagery exercises, the *Question Mark Exercise* is quite simple. And like most imagery exercises, it is very fast, by which I mean it is short and its effects happen quickly.

So, find yourself now sitting in the Pharaoh's Posture, eyes closed, forming an even and regular cycle of breathing, breathing out through the mouth and breathing in through the nose. And now, as you form this even and regular cycle of breathing, find yourself breathing out a long, slow exhalation, and breathing in briefly, three times. You know that you are doing the exercise to start the day with freshness and that it is taking a few seconds.

Now see in front of you a silhouette or profile form of yourself, and you see you are in the shape of a question mark. If you can, notice the look on your face. Now, breathe out one time slowly, and see yourself turning towards you. And as you turn towards you, see yourself becoming an exclamation mark. See, sense, and feel what happens as you complete this experience, and if you can, notice the expression on your face.

After finishing, breathe out and open your eyes.

How do you feel? Do you notice any sensations, movement, or changes? Is there anything different about the way you look? Is there any difference between being in the question mark and being in the exclamation mark? Some of you may notice that in going from the first to the second, you become taller and feel lighter, that your posture becomes straighter, that the expression on your face changes from one that may have been a little gloomy or downcast to one that is brighter. Many kinds of changes may be experienced.

Now, if changes occurred, keep in mind that with this exercise you now have the possibility of making some shifts in your life very quickly. In the course of a day, you may notice changes in your usual response to events. Keep in mind too whether the imaginal changes you noticed on one day occur the next day. Become observant of yourself; this is an act of remembering yourself. You may make notes in a little breast pocket notebook used for this purpose.

Or, you might not have experienced anything. That is okay. Every person is different. We all come to ourselves in our own time. Keep doing the exercise during a 21-day period. See what happens. Remember, put your goals aside. Concentrate on your intention and your practice.

The Centering Exercise

Here is a second exercise to start the day with vigor and confidence.

Again, this exercise is short.

Close your eyes and breathe out three times slowly. Know you are doing the exercise to start the day with vigor and that it is taking only a few seconds.

Now see yourself becoming a dot in the center of a circle. See, sense, and feel what happens. Experience this momentarily, then breathe out and open your eyes.

Notice what happens to you and how you feel. Do you find yourself easily becoming this dot in the circle? Is there a sense of centering that takes place when you do this? Is there some resistance to doing it? If there is resistance, it means either that you may not be ready to do the exercise or, perhaps, that you do not relate to it.

When people first do this particular exercise, some of them say "I need more time; this is too quick." Such a response tells us about our relationship to time, which is often the habitual one of either trying to extend it or of being captured by it and becoming enslaved to it. In this exercise, we seem almost not to need time.

If the brevity of the exercise makes you feel uncomfortable, extend the time to give yourself only a few more seconds. Remember, though, the more you extend the time, the less power the imagery has. I know that some of us naturally take more time in the thinking process. It is especially important for those of you who have this characteristic to expend the effort to do the exercises quickly. You want the habitual mind to have as little opportunity as possible to interject itself into the non-habitual process of imagery.

How to Use These Exercises

I recommend that in the morning you do one of these exercises or one that you devise before doing any other daily activity, other than going to the bathroom to urinate. Any other activity that you normally would do – bathing, shaving, defecating, eating – should take place after the exercise. By starting the day with the exercise, you are starting a habitual day non-habitually. You are bringing a new attitude into the day and influencing the day you are about to live in a new way – which is why the man I described above tried so vigorously at first to approach all his early morning routines with awareness and choice and why he kept to his early morning imagery exercise.

Some people tell me that they find it hard to remember to do an exercise first thing. They explain that their habits are such that they get up, do their daily routines and then go to work, more or less on automatic pilot, and that doing the exercise just does not come to mind. If you are such person, here is what you can do: When you open your eyes, the first thing to do is to say the word "remember" and/or the phrase "I am here." By saying "I am here" or "remember," something special takes place because you are putting yourself into *this* life and you are acknowledging, at the same time, a relationship with the invisible reality. Remember that "remember" reminds you to put yourself together and "I am" invites your special connection to the invisible reality. As God said to Moses: "I AM THAT I AM" you can also say, "I AM *is* here."

As for the broader applications of these exercises, both are calming, centering, and restorative. For example, you can use the centering exercise to become centered and focused whenever you are feeling out of sorts, experiencing a sense of imbalance, or feeling at odds with yourself for whatever reason. You can also use it to bring yourself into an unfamiliar place – physically, emotionally, mentally, socially – that you have not habitually taken on and to integrate it often instantaneously.

In general, I also recommend that you do either exercise when you come home from your job or at the end of whatever efforts you go through during the day. Doing the exercises helps to revive you from all the stresses, stimuli and shocks of the day that you encounter. I understand that sometimes the activities of your day may not be completed until well into the evening. If this is the case, I recommend that you do an exercise around the time of sundown, if possible.

Beyond this, you can use these exercises anytime you feel overwhelmed, anytime you feel any sort of distress in your life, anytime you feel overworked, or anytime you are feeling a sense of emergency. Each exercise will calm you and restore you. They bring you back to who you are, free of the heavy shadows of the world that cloud your vision and behavior and deplete your energies. By doing these exercises, you are following a kabbalistic prescription for taking charge of your inner state of being, an absolute necessity for making a turn toward Spirit.

Chapter 4.

ABOUT BALANCE AND PATIENCE

You will come to notice that the pages immediately ahead are peppered with the words "balance" and its opposite, "imbalance." More importantly, you will see the *idea* of balance is central to understanding the kabbalistic perspective on health. In kabbalistic thought, balance means a coming into order and integration; and balance, order, and integration, taken together, equals healing. Again and again, you will observe that I recommend mental exercises that restore balance – sometimes by righting an imbalance, sometimes by transforming the remembrance of an event. Whatever the approach, the idea of wholeness, of balance, underlies the recommendation.

There are four elements to balance – proportion, measure, rhythm, and pace; and, contrariwise, four opposite elements to imbalance – disproportion, immoderation, arrhythmia, and irregularity. I am confident that most of us are familiar with all four elements of imbalance, having experienced them at one time or another in our thoughts, feelings, and behavior. When out of balance we are not happy and in charge of ourselves and have to "put ourselves together" again. Our experience shows that Kabbalah's principle of balance is sound. In terms of health, where imbalance prevails, there is vulnerability. Physically, emotionally, spiritually, when something is out of whack, the damage will become worse unless it is corrected.

A number of people who come to see me suffer from disturbances brought on by breakdowns in the regular rhythms and patterns of their lives. Valerie was a vivid example. She was a vivacious young woman, who worked hard and functioned well at her steady job. She lived with her boyfriend, whose life seemed more irregular and less settled than hers. One day she returned home from work to find that he had moved out, leaving only a note. She was devastated. The shock sent her into a state of disorientation. She developed a cardiac arrhythmia. Then she developed a mysterious illness that was never fully diagnosed. It left her drained and depleted to the point that she was unable to perform her job, which she eventually lost.

Valerie had only minimal resources to sustain her. She was thoroughly frightened. Her pattern of life was severely interrupted, replaced by an arrhythmic life of stops and starts: intermittent bouts of cardiac arrhythmia, sometimes necessitating trips to the emergency room; intermittent interviews in her attempts to find a job; intermittent bouts of illness; and persistent disagreements with others.

She came to me, hoping that I would be able to show her how to restore some order to her life. As she put it, she wanted her sense of balance restored. She felt that once this happened, she would be able to deal with all her difficulties. She wanted to be able to step back from the sense that she was standing "at the edge of a cliff" (her words).

In my view, Valerie fundamentally suffered from a broken heart that was reflected in and by the cardiac arrhythmia. I proposed that she use mental imagery to reverse the arrhythmia and to create a sense of inner balance. First, we worked on the arrhythmia with an exercise to restore the regular rhythm of her heart. Next, we worked on her sense of standing on a cliff with an exercise to root her to level ground. She soon found herself firmly back on her feet.

Patience is related to all four elements of balance in that it requires proportion, measure, rhythm, and pace. Kabbalistically speaking, patience is a highly sought virtue. To be patient is to wait, to be able to mentally insert a wedge between a linked stimulus and response and so place a stop on repetitive, habitual, often impatient behavior. Patience gives you a moment to assess, step back from the brink, and bring yourself back into balance.

The ability to restrain oneself is echoed in Western spirituality through a practice called deeds, or *mitzvoth* in Hebrew. There are 613 of these deeds or activities, and 365 of them (the number of days in a year) are connected with the use of our musculature, the muscles being the physical expression of will. The idea is that we restrain our will to stop an impulsive or destructive action and turn our energy in a constructive or creative direction – to use will in a directly beneficial way. Patience, then, is the mental reflection of the restraint of will.

The chapters ahead will provide many examples of exercises to restore balance and patience in particular situations. Here I want to offer a set of seven exercises to help bring about balance and patience in general. In this society, subject as we are to inputs of all types and a virtually unending need to schedule our lives, a spirit of balance – so central to our health – and an attitude of patience rarely come by themselves. These exercises take their inspiration from the story of Job, renowned for his patience in the face of seemingly unending, catastrophic loss.

The intention of all seven exercises is to be centered, balanced and patient. The time for each exercise is a few seconds in the morning and early evening (between 5-6 pm) for up to 21 days. Some of you may not understand the biblical references in some of the exercises, so do the exercises with which you are most comfortable. If you find yourself curious about the exercises that are not clear to you, turn to the Book of Job, where the story of Job makes everything clear.

The Job Exercises

Close your eyes. Breathe out three times slowly. Know you are doing a Job exercise to be centered, balanced and patient, and that it is taking a few seconds.
Live, as Job, the bet made between God and Satan: that you can be turned from faith in the certainty of the reality of God. Breathe out and open your eyes.

Close your eyes. Breathe out one time slowly. Know you are doing a Job exercise to be centered, balanced and patient, and that it is taking a few seconds.
Know and live your loss as Job, not understanding why, but staying in the moment, accepting and responding. Don't accept to remain sad. Breathe out and open your eyes.

Close your eyes. Breathe out three times slowly. Know that you are doing a Job exercise to be centered, balanced and patient, and that it is taking a few seconds.

See and sense yourself resisting the suggestions of the false comforters who have come to visit you, seemingly as friends. Don't become self-blaming or critical of God. Breathe out once. Know, now, who and what is a true friend. Breathe out and open your eyes.

Close your eyes. Breathe out three times slowly. Know you are doing a Job exercise to be centered, balanced and patient, and that it is taking a few seconds.

Hear the still small voice issuing forth out of the whirlwind, confirming your faith in God. Hear what this voice has to tell you. What do you see now?

Breathe out and open your eyes.

Close your eyes. Breathe out three times slowly. Know you are doing a Job exercise to be centered, balanced and patient, and that it is taking a few seconds.

See and know, as Job, that you understand what Moses experienced at the burning bush. Breathe out and open your eyes.

Close your eyes. Breathe out three times slowly. Know you are doing a Job exercise to be centered, balanced and patient, and that it is taking a few seconds.

See, feel, and sense all that you have lost being restored to you. Breathe out once. Know why the physical disease has not disappeared. Breathe out and open your eyes.

Close your eyes. Breathe out three times slowly. Know you are doing a Job exercise to be centered, balanced and patient, and that it is taking a few seconds.

Feel, as Satan, the loss of God's realm, having fallen from there. Breathe out three times. Know and live why God has to retrieve Satan as a reason for the creation of the world. Breathe out and open your eyes.

Chapter 5.

MALADIES OF EVERYDAY LIFE:
ANXIETY AND PAIN

During the course of an ordinary day, many people experience different situations about which they become anxious. Will you meet a deadline at work? Will you be able to meet your friend on time? Maybe you have a regular dental appointment just to have your teeth cleaned – but you feel anxious. Many things that happen – or don't happen – can elicit anxiety, and virtually everyone has his or her anxious "hot spots." For some people, every day can be filled with experiences of anxiety; for others, anxiety can be overwhelming.

Pain of varying severity is another common touchstone of life. Perhaps you have a sore muscle from running or from shoveling snow. Perhaps you fell on an arm or leg racing to catch a bus. Perhaps you have something more serious, like back pain or a strained hamstring. Aches and pains come and go, bothering some people more than others. In some cases, pain can disable us, keep us in bed or away from the everyday activities that give meaning to our lives.

If we see anxiety and pain for what they are – the manifestations of imbalances in our lives – we know that we need more than pills to deal with them. Otherwise, if we do not see the reality of anxiety and pain, and the signals they are sending to investigate what the imbalance is about, we tend to find our lives moving into deeper and deeper imbalance.

60

Kabbalah tells us that there is no escaping such experiences as anxiety and pain (or frustration and disappointment, which we will not consider here) – nor should there be. The point is not simply that life contains hard times – though this is certainly true – but rather, that these hard times bring us lessons that we need. They tell us there is an imbalance in our lives that we are to correct. And what might be the source of the imbalance? The key kabbalistic principle – that beliefs (concepts, images) give birth to experience – tells us that the source is a false belief.

The story of Sarah, a highly successful woman who had gone through some rough times and who was suffering from a high level of anxiety when she came to see me, puts all this in perspective.

Sarah had made and lost a fortune over the years. When I saw her, she had rallied back from difficult circumstances and was on the brink of a financial breakthrough with a number of projects that she had been nurturing simultaneously. As this breakthrough was about to happen, Sarah received a job offer in a completely unrelated field, one that would put her in the public eye. The offer was very attractive, and she felt tempted to take it. She asked a number of people close to her for their opinions about what her decision should be, and after having heard many different perspectives, she came to see me in a frazzled state.

We did an imagery exercise to relieve anxiety – *Finding the Room of Silence* – which I describe extensively later. In this exercise, she saw herself in a room standing in front of the anxiety. She then turned her back on the anxiety and went through a door into another room, then through a door in that room to yet another room. As she went on, she related that she had been calling person after person asking for advice, and becoming increasingly unnerved when they gave it to her. Finally, she found her room of silence, which she could calmly explore as she wished to find her own answer.

As Sarah was a spiritually-oriented person, I set her predicament within the framework of the 10 Commandments, the universal moral laws of balance. She was clearly seeking an outside authority to tell her right from wrong. She complained that she was feeling alone and needed the help of others. I explained to her that whenever we turn from the invisible reality, we feel alone. For the invisible reality, Sarah had substituted the visible reality in the form of her many advisors. There was little value, I said, in putting the visible reality between herself and the invisible. In effect, she was going against the first law of balance: "Don't put any god before God."

She said that made a lot of sense, since she had been seeking answers from outside rather than from within herself. She saw that she was shortchanging and ultimately sabotaging herself by shifting her own authority to others. In fact, by surrendering her power, she had let herself be deflected from her creative pursuits.

Along with this new understanding of her efficacy came a sense of new-found power and relief from anxiety. She turned down the job offer and completed the work that was where her heart really was. Since then, whenever anxiety has come back to her, she has been able to calm herself easily by using her imagery exercise.

Sarah's dilemma was no different from the dilemma virtually all of us face in our lives. Almost all of us abdicate our power and turn to outside authorities, believing that they know more about us than we do. This is a false belief, and to the degree that we cling to it, we create an imbalance in ourselves – which can show itself as anxiety.

As we shall see, and as I might have noted to Sarah had she not been open to seeing anxiety in the spiritual framework of the 10 Commandments, there is another false belief that always gives rise to anxiety.

In kabbalistic thought, if we are to grow, we use the experiences that disturb us to learn the ways in which we are imbalanced so that we can then right ourselves. In doing this, we obviously fulfill the general principle of Kabbalah to maintain our health so that we are better prepared to open ourselves to receiving the input of Spirit.

In the assorted imagery exercises that I recommend for anxiety and pain, I include exercises that primarily are intended to quell the symptoms and exercises that allow us to reach the imbalance fueling them. Like the exercises in the previous chapters, these exercises are brief, and they demonstrate our remarkable ability to restore ourselves emotionally and physically through the power of our directed imaginal experiences.

How to Confront Anxiety

The example of Sarah shows us that we experience anxiety as a response to life's tumult and uncertainty. At its worst, anxiety can be crippling. It possesses us by constricting our emotions and our bodies. In the mind, anxiety brings forth its companion vipers of worry, fear, and apprehension. In the body, it strangles the breath and disturbs the natural rhythms of the heart and intestinal tract.

The danger is that the turbulent feelings of anxiety obscure the lesson it carries. The sufferer needs to acknowledge the presence of the experience and avoid entanglement in its symptoms. Only then can the meaning of the experience become clear. In other words, learn to step back to observe what's going on, and you shall make *discoveries* about your situation that may even surprise you.

To translate the cryptic language of anxiety, we ask, "Anxiety about what?" If I ask you, "What are you anxious about?" I can assure you that you will give me an answer that concerns a future event. Speaking of the future *always* represents a mirage or an illusion – a fabricated "reality" that doesn't exist, but nonetheless is treated as though it were a presently existing reality. Future talk can *never* be about anything other than a potential or a probability. In kabbalistic terms, the future belongs to God. In Sarah's case, it was through worry about the future that she allocated her authority to others, stumbling from one false belief to another.

If you probe further into a concern about the future, you will find that the worry is always linked with *survival*, broadly understood. You may be anxious about a test in school, about an interview for a new job, about whether the party you give will be a success, and so forth. In all such instances, failure means that your life will take a turn for the worse. It will not be the life you want.

At its base, anxiety is a necessary disruption of our equilibrium. A situation occurs and impels us to relinquish our falsely established notions of unruffled safety to the clear perception that there is no safety in the man-made world. In an upheaval of anxiety, we can either succumb to the anxiety, which means that we collapse to some small or large degree, or we can listen to its message. Anxiety provides us with a needed message, that we are in a state of imbalance, that in our habits or our beliefs we are following a false path. In the reversing of these habits or beliefs, we can discover the glimmer of some essential truth of ourselves. We then return to life in an entirely new way.

Simply understanding the intimate connection between anxiety and the future we can never know often helps loosen the hold of anxiety. At other times, we may need to deal directly with the state of anxiety itself, as did Sarah.

There are many expressions of anxiety and many ways to deal with it. Here is a sampling of exercises that I have gleaned from people suffering with anxiety who came to see me and who devised their own imaginal ways to deal with it. Imagery is the shared social language of the world. It is the language of cooperation, the language that binds us together. So one person's image may be effective for many other people, because it is an expression of something we share in common.

Obviously, the exercises that follow by no means exhaust the possibilities. The realm of imagination is a limitless one; we are all individuals with creativity, and there is no end to the creative possibilities of the imagination.

The Room of Silence Exercise

Close your eyes and breathe out slowly three times. Remember, just the act of long, slow exhalations and brief inhalations will reduce anxiety. You are doing The Room of Silence Exercise to quell or stop anxiety, and it takes up to 15 seconds.

Imagine yourself in a room together with the feeling of anxiety. Turn your back on the anxiety and find the door to the right out of that room to go into another room. If there is noise/cacophony go through that door to your right, eventually coming to a room of silence where the noise has stopped. When you come to that room of silence, look around and see what you discover there. You may have to go through door after door after door in each room until eventually you come to the room of silence and when you do, the anxiety is gone. See what you discover in that room. And when you are finished, you can breathe out and open your eyes.

The reason I ask you to discover what you may see in that room of silence is because, by itself, it may serve you as a reminder of how you can be free of anxiety. The next time that the anxiety comes, you may not have to go through all the rooms. Just by recalling what was in the room of silence may be enough to stop the anxiety. It will remind you of a time you shed the anxiety and left it behind. The memory is both powerful and pleasant and can stop the anxiety state almost instantaneously.

What you find in the room of silence is what you find. There is no predicting what will be there. What is there is what you need. In kabbalistic terms, it is what the language of image carries to you from the invisible universe. Use it as you wish.

A young man imagined himself going through various rooms until he found the room of silence, and discovered there a picture on the wall, a picture of a shepherd with lambs. I asked him to go into that picture and become the shepherd. He led the lambs into a meadow, where he saw a valley into which he descended, and there he felt much calmer, more peaceful, and found a person who was very kind to him and with whom he could discuss the anxiety in a clear, free and open way.

As some readers may know through experience, we have inner guides with whom we can make contact. These inner guides are real beings who exist for us in the inner-dimensional realities that we discover. They are there to help us and protect us. They give us answers to life and provide us with information about how to approach life in ways that differ from our habitual practices. The person the young man discovered in the meadow was his inner guide. After discussing his fears with his guide, the young man returned feeling much better than he did when he had started.

The young man's discovery of the picture is a good example of the discoveries you may make when you do an imagery exercise. You may find new things for yourself, new possibilities in the form of images or people. Any discovery of this sort is an opening that allows you to go deeper into yourself to expand your consciousness, broaden your outlook, and come to new understandings, new revelations about yourself.

Like the young man, accept these opportunities. If you see a picture, enter it; if you come upon an exotic plant, enter into it; if you come across a character from a novel or a movie or even someone you've never seen or met before – even an angel – speak to it.

The possibilities are open and endless in this kind of process, and they are there to bring help to you.

As you do this exercise, as an example, when you exit the tent, the day is very sunny and very bright, and the sky is quite blue and even cloudless. The scene is showing us that the anxiety has been replaced by a sense of inner peacefulness and placidity. As this is imagination anything may happen.

Now, three very short exercises to relieve anxiety and make us quiet so we can discover sources of anxiety. Choose whichever exercise works for you.

The Desert Storm Exercise

Close your eyes and breathe out three times slowly. Know that you are doing The Desert Storm Exercise to remove anxiety and that it is taking 15 to 30 seconds.

See yourself entering a desert, carrying a backpack which is an enfolded tent, and as you are moving along in the desert, you begin to see dark clouds forming in front of you. A stiff, strong wind begins to rise. The sand begins to kick up, clouds are building, and the wind is increasing. You see that this storm is moving towards you. You know that this is the storm of anxiety.

Now, you take the backpack off your back and you set up your tent. You hook the ends of the tent strings around the stakes and drive the stakes into the earth. As the storm is getting closer and closer, you hear the sound of the wind, the sound of the sand. You open the flap, crawl inside, and are there in a tent full of blue light.

And as you are inside, the wind and sand hit the tent, and you hear the sound outside, and you are sitting safely inside a tent filled with blue light, and the wind and the sand pass, and outside the tent, it becomes silent. When you hear the silence, you know the anxiety is gone, and now you can open the flap of the tent and come out, and you see and sense what you feel when you exit the tent. And when you are ready, you breathe out and open your eyes.

The American Indian Exercise (originated by Native American tribes)

Close your eyes, and breathe out three times slowly. Know you are doing The American Indian Exercise to remove anxiety and that it takes only seconds.

See yourself on the seashore. The sky is clear. See and feel anxiety abiding in you like a stone or a rock. Let the water and wind erode this rock, washing and blowing away the particles that remain after the erosion. See, sense, and know that when all the particles are gone, the anxiety has gone as well. And now breathe out and open your eyes.

The Elevator Exercise

Close your eyes, and breathe out three times slowly. Know that you are doing The Elevator Exercise to remove anxiety and that it takes a few seconds.

See yourself entering an elevator at the 15th floor. Press the button that says "G" for ground floor. The doors close, the elevator begins to descend. You see the panel of the floor numbers on the wall of the elevator. As you pass each floor, the floor numbers light up, 14, 13, 12, 11, 10, and so on, and when you reach the ground floor, the doors open and you emerge from the elevator anxiety-free. Breathe out and open your eyes.

The Net of Anxiety Exercise

Close your eyes and breathe out three times slowly. Know that you are doing The Net of Anxiety Exercise to relieve anxiety and that it takes a few seconds.

See, sense, and feel the net of anxiety

wrapped tightly around you. Breathe out one time slowly and remove the net, knowing that as you do, the anxiety disappears. Then, breathe out and open your eyes.

How to Confront Pain

Pain and anxiety are related to each other, anxiety being the emotional form of pain and pain the physical form of anxiety.

As is anxiety, pain is a necessary component of life in the kabbalistic perspective. It is the signal of human error, and no one is free of committing errors. Our errors are experienced as pain or guilt, which can be felt on three levels: on the mental level as doubt, on the emotional level as anxiety or guilt, and on the physical level as a disturbing discomfort. Thus, pain signals an imbalance in living registered on any one or combination of the three levels. From the spiritual perspective, when we are in balance, in equilibrium, we do not experience pain. Ergo, it is natural to experience pain, but it is not normal. Natural refers to what is conditioned or reflexive in us. Normal means what is a balanced, sober, in-charge response that is free of habitual conditioning. The same holds true for all signs of distress.

The initial experience of physical pain is a benefit to us because it shows us that there is a disorder somewhere in our lives manifesting itself in our bodies. But once pain has made us stop and become watchers of ourselves, once it has alerted us to what is necessary, we want to dispel it. We do not want it to remain with us, because it eventually becomes a corrosive factor. It erodes our lives, depletes us of energy, and has the effect of pushing us to feel depressed.

In the English language, the etymological root of the word "pain" also gives rise to the word "punishment." The association of pain and punishment is meaningful. You can see the connection in two ways. In one perspective, we experience the punishment of pain because we have committed an error in living. From another perspective, perhaps closer to the truth, the pain we feel is the punishment we bring upon ourselves for committing an error. Somewhere within us, we know that we have erred.

In Sanskrit, I should mention, the root of pain gives rise to "purification," another significant association, as we shall see in the first exercise to reduce pain called *The Prisoner of Pain.*

The key point to remember is that pain is a message asking for our help. We should not run away from pain but rather recognize it as a call to examine where our lives are out of balance. It is sometimes difficult for people to see that pain is an expression of imbalance. Say you are driving your car, waiting at a stoplight, and a car driven by a drunk hits the rear of your car hard enough that you knock your head on the steering wheel. You can say that the resulting pain in your head has nothing to do with an imbalance in you. After all, you didn't ram your car into the car in front of you; a drunk rammed his car into your car. I would say that you may have needed to have some sense knocked into you. Whatever may be the case, the possible meaning of your experience is certainly worth further investigation.

Here is an imagery exercise that may help in perceiving the error behind pain.

The Prisoner of Pain Exercise

Close your eyes and breathe out and in three times slowly, knowing that you are doing The Prisoner of Pain Exercise to end your punishment of pain and that it takes 10 to 15 seconds.

See, sense, and feel how the pain is connected with some significant person or event. Breathe out three times. Do whatever is necessary to get rid of the pain or to quiet the pain. Breathe out three times. Feel and know how the pain has passed beyond the meaning of punishment to purification. Breathe out three times. See a golden blue light pouring on you outside and inside. Breathe out three times. See yourself not accepting being a prisoner of pain.

Breathe out and open your eyes.

Do this exercise whenever you feel the pain, until the pain stops recurring.

The Sander Exercise

There are many exercises for physical pain, partly because there are many ways we individually experience it. To identify the individual way you experience pain, ask yourself what your pain looks like. Most people who do this see the pain clearly as an image. And when you see it as an image, then you can deal with it in an effective way.

The story behind *The Sander Exercise*, devised by one of my patients, is a good example.

Alice was in severe pain, and she hoped I could help her get rid of it. I asked her to tell me what the pain looked like. She concentrated for a few seconds and reported that the pain was a black rock with many jagged edges. I asked her, "How could you get rid of such an object?" She thought for a moment. "I'm going to get rid of it by taking a sander and sanding down the jagged edges. And once I do it, I'm going to throw the rock away." So, she did just that – establishing her breathing and her intention, she used a sander on her rock of pain, and the pain did go away.

For some people, doing the exercise once is sufficient. Others may need to repeat it at the three set times a day for a day or two, as well as when the pain may recur.

The Crystal Exercise

One imagery exercise that I think might be very useful for relieving pain, particularly severe pain, is *The Crystal Exercise*.

Close your eyes and see yourself holding a beautiful crystal, a clear crystal that has no blemishes. You are holding its ends. And you put this crystal over an area of pain in your body, wherever it is, and see a beam of green light coming from above. The green light shines directly through the crystal and then diffuses itself from there into the area of the pain, dispersing and dissolving the pain.

Sense and feel what happens, and when you are ready, breathe out and open your eyes.

Some readers will have noticed that at the start of this exercise, I did not say to set your breaths and intention. This is not an oversight. Because you are in pain, you may not want to spend any time quieting yourself. You just want to take care of the pain immediately. Of course, you may breathe out and in one time before you do this exercise, to achieve a moment of quietness and to focus on the exercise. But you also can just close your eyes and do the exercise.

The Red Circle Exercise

This is an extremely short exercise provided by my student Ruth.

See your pain, and put a red circle around it to contain it.
See and feel what happens.

A successful exercise to remove pain does not necessarily mean that the pain will stay gone. It may. But it may not. There are certain times in our lives when a difficulty we experience has its own rhythm. Anxiety is like that. Also, pain is like that – it has its own rhythm. If the pain returns, you do the successful exercise then and there. You do not have to think about doing the exercise three times a day at set times. You simply do the exercise when the difficulty occurs.

It is likely that each person will respond differently to each of the pain exercises I have suggested. One may work better than others. Some people may find that none of them is strongly effective. Do not worry. There is always a possibility for everyone, always a way to find something for everybody. You will find the possibility that works for you by asking yourself what your pain looks like and then building an exercise on the basis of that image, a simple process we discuss in "Notes on How to Create Your Own Imagery," at the end of the book.

Chapter 6.

MONEY WORRIES, MONEY TRAPS

Whether we leave for work in the morning or stay at home to raise our children, many of us have a concern in common: money. Do we have enough for our bills? Will we be able to afford the vacation we want? How will we accumulate the funds to put our children through college? Where can we find the money to help one of our parents, who all of a sudden needs a medical procedure that is extremely expensive? Are we putting away enough for our own future? These concerns are generally referred to as "money worries." We live in a society where money helps dictate the options before us and is a constant focus of our attention and worry. How can we navigate the "money worries" that often arise in such a society?

There is a second set of money concerns, which perhaps is not as clear as "money worries." I call them "money traps." These concerns arise from our attitudes toward money, from not properly distinguishing between needs and desires, and from using money either selfishly or in a spendthrift manner to establish an image of ourselves. Profligacy is a common money trap. How can we circumvent these money mazes and other issues surrounding money that often bring such unhappiness to us and sometimes corrupt many of our relations with other people?

The old quip goes, "You can't be too rich or too thin." Kabbalah has little to say about thinness, except for the one key point that health is more important than achieving a standard called thinness.

But with regard to money, Kabbalah has much to offer in helping us put our attitudes toward money in perspective and avoid the various money snares around us, many of which are intensified, by our consumerist, money-driven society.

Our starting place is a basic idea of Kabbalah that I set out in the introduction – that if we are in accord with the invisible universe, it brings us a life of abundance. As I further explained, abundance does not simply mean money; it means self-fulfillment, loving relationships, spiritual freedom. Money can certainly be *part* of these conditions, and it can be *part* of the abundance of life that we are promised if we keep ourselves open to Spirit. Being a *part* of means that it does not split itself off from the other values of abundance. Money simply becomes an energy of exchange between people, a means towards something, not an end in itself. In Kabbalah, the guiding idea with regard to money – as with all our behavior – is to be moderate, which in this case means being sober about money, and being neither too rich nor too poor.

Does this mean that once we put ourselves in accord with the invisible reality – a process we aim toward continuously throughout life – it will shower us with the financial sufficiency we need? Yes. We are always receiving what we need as well as what is necessary to face as a challenge to overcome from our friend, the invisible reality. But what we need is not equivalent to what we may want.

The failure to make the distinction between need and want leads us to the most pervasive money trap of contemporary life – the bottomless well of want. We may want a 60" television set, but do we really need it? Admittedly, we sometimes want because the natural tendency of our conditioning is to desire. But society today reinforces this natural tendency through a destructive belief with which we are all infected – something I learned from Dr. Robert Rhondell Gibson: the belief that the purpose of life is to reach the non-disturbed state in which we always experience pleasure and avoid experiencing pain. This leads to a strongly conditioned tendency to remain unsatisfied, even if we have at hand everything we had wanted, because now we want something else! This tendency leads to the "greed factor," always wanting more, better, and different.

All around us, this bottomless wanting is made to seem entirely natural. It is the way we are told to live. Indeed, after 9/11, President Bush told us that what the ordinary citizen should do to help the country is, "Keep shopping." It seems as if there is no other way to respond to an event that stunned the nation, bringing grief and fear: "Keep shopping!"

However, there is an easy way to tell the difference between want and need if we are honest with ourselves. You walk by the shoe store and are taken by a beautiful pair of shoes. You know you have several pairs in your closet. Do you want this pair? Acknowledge your desire for them and then ask, "Do I need them?" The answer will almost invariably be "no." When it is "yes," the need is certainly valid.

Now, there are those of us who might feel the need for something in order to feel better. This feeling is a want disguised as a need – the want being "to feel better." Indeed, we can observe that the fashion industry's very existence is predicated on both a woman's attempt to overcome depressed feelings and a man's attempt to prop up his self-image (which we more properly term "vanity") through shopping.

Spendthriftiness is one money trap; miserliness is another. They are both common. Each is a disproportion that has to be avoided. Profligacy, with its wasteful, unnecessary spending, makes us unmindful of the possibility of lean years ahead and of forces of nature that may disrupt our economic lives, sometimes without warning. Miserliness, stinginess, and the withholding of funds, make us ungenerous, unloving, incapable of sharing, withholding, and unable to effect deep, affectionate relationships.

The story of a young woman who came to see me illustrates another money trap – a variation of spendthriftiness, but not for the self. This young woman, who made a modest income as a secretary for a nonprofit organization, was always giving to good causes, always emptying her pockets to beggars on the street. At work, she regularly used her own funds to pay for many of her supplies (pens, pads, ink for her printer, and so forth) because she wanted to "spare" the organization the cost so that it could use the saved money for those in need. After it became known at her office that she was buying her own supplies, she was forbidden to do so. This edict brought the young woman to see me. She was deeply unhappy. No one appreciated her generosity, she said. Somewhere between tears and anger, she cried out: "How could people be so mean?"

We took up her being too generous, a quality that created trouble elsewhere in her life. To find the *balance* for herself, I gave her *The Sweet Fruit Exercise*.

The Sweet Fruit Exercise

Close your eyes. Breathe out three times slowly. Know you are doing The Sweet Fruit Exercise with the intention of becoming frugal and that it is taking a few seconds.

See yourself in a large candy shop. Sense the excitement of wanting to taste these delicious morsels. As you reach to take one, see it turn into your favorite fruit. Take it and eat it, feeling satisfied.

Breathe out and open your eyes, knowing you are curbing your spending.

I recommended that she do the exercise for 21 days – early in the morning, before each expenditure, and before bed. The success of the exercise for her became a turning point in her life, not only for her relationship to her work, but for her life in general. Put simply, she no longer needed to be overly generous to others to feel satisfied.

Even as we live in a web of money, the Kabbalah tells us and teaches us that life is not about money, despite the fact that almost all of us are required to earn a living by the sweat of our brows. The spiritual approach to the subject of money is to become frugal, a virtue defined as not making *unnecessary* expenditures. We distinguish between necessary and unnecessary by distinguishing between need and want. We are neither to be too rich nor too poor. We are to follow the tenth law of balance – the 10th Commandment not to covet. We are not to compare ourselves to others (prelude to envy and jealousy), and we are to fight against the tide of the greed factor so dominant in the mass consciousness of the world (See Chapter 13).

Spiritual understanding means we cannot serve two masters at the same time. We cannot have our eyes on material possession and acquisition (usually at the expense of others) – thus serving Mammon – and also have an eye turned toward Spirit.

To resolve misguided ideas about money and worries that we will not have the financial where-withal to care for ourselves and those we love, we acknowledge that we are connected to the energy of the universe and that we live within its sustenance. If we live in accord with the principles of Spirit, the universe will see to it that we have enough to main-tain the basics of life – food, shelter, and clothing – and will not let us fall prey to the clutches of Mammon and, more broadly, the whole arena of idolatry.

Here are two mental imagery exercises that can help us obtain the money we need.

The Stream of Money Exercise

Close your eyes. Breathe out three times slowly. Know you are doing The Stream of Money Exercise to connect with the energy of the universe, and that it takes a few seconds.

See and know that you are connected with the energy of the universe. See a beam of white heavenly light come down toward you to confirm that connection. As the light gets closer and closer, see within it a stream of money that flows over and around you. Breathe out one time. Sense and know the endless sustenance the universe is bestowing on you just for the asking.

Breathe out and open your eyes.

The Hot Air Balloon Exercise (created by Dr. Lydia Craigmyle)

Close your eyes. Breathe out three times slowly. Know you are doing The Hot Air Balloon Exercise to bring to yourself the money you need and that it takes 15 seconds.

Look up to the upper right in a cloudless blue sky. See there a black dot. See the dot descending toward you. As it gets closer and closer, you see that it is a brightly colored, gaily decorated hot air balloon. It lands on the earth to the right of you. You reach into the basket and take out an envelope with your name on the front. Open the envelope and find inside a check made out to you in the amount you need, signed by the Heavenly Father (or Power). Take the check for yourself and see the balloon ascend the way it came, until it becomes the black dot at the upper right and then disappears.

Then breathe out and open your eyes.

Do this exercise each morning and at sundown for 21 days. If you receive what you need before then, you can stop the exercise.

Here is an exercise for miserliness and its variations.

The Beggar Exercise

Close your eyes, breathe out three times slowly. Know you are doing The Beggar Exercise with the intention of becoming frugal and that it takes a few seconds.

See yourself walking in a very rich neighborhood. Suddenly, you come upon a beggar who asks you for money. Place a coin or two in his hand, no more. Wish him/her well and walk on. Then, breathe out and open your eyes.

Do this exercise three times a day for 21 days – early in the morning, at late afternoon, and before bed.

Chapter 7.

WHEN WE LOSE OUR FOOTING: SELF-DOUBT, INDECISIVENESS, DISQUIETING FEELINGS

In the course of a day, we face many challenges. We tend to have various habitual ways of dealing with them, though usually the same challenges keep reoccurring – a sign that our habitual approach is not fully adequate. The more we open to the universe by following the path of Kabbalah, the more we can see these struggles for what they are – part of coming to grips with the process of learning what it truly is to be an adult, a task that demands much pain and work. Along the way, there can be many pitfalls, most of which tend to be of our own making, either intentionally or unwittingly. In any case, pitfalls are unavoidable. They provide the crucible in which we can reshape, refine, and revamp our lives, so that we live as aware human beings on this planet.

Life's pitfalls and disappointments are both small and large: the promotion we hoped for goes to someone else; the investment we made fails; people we care for treat us badly; we realize that we have treated someone badly; someone we love dies. None of these is extraordinary. They are familiar, everyday pains of life. Yet each and every one is enough to send us stumbling.

We lose our footing. We begin to doubt ourselves. We become indecisive. We have feelings that thoroughly upset us – feelings of anger or hostility or even rage – and we cannot shake them loose.

Our task is to face these challenges and struggles as opportunities – dramas that can make us more mature, more securely responsive to life in its variety. They don't happen by chance, but allow us opportunities to make corrections for the errors we seek to overcome to achieve maturity. In this chapter, I deal with three inner experiences that can throw us off balance: self-doubt, indecisiveness, and disquieting feelings. Note how we use imagery – the language of Spirit – to resolve them while simultaneously strengthening our spirit.

Often these feelings are habitual, constants in our lives. In these cases, we seek not simply to resolve the experiences when they occur, but to free ourselves from the grips of their habitual occurrence. This is simple enough to say and, as you will find, simple enough to do. But many people do not see themselves as free. Some say, "You can't teach an old dog new tricks." Others say, "It's because of the way I was raised, and I can't change that." Some insist, "It's not a habit; it's my experiences in the world that lead me to react as I do." Remember, in the kabbalistic perspective, you are free to reshape yourselves. Imagery is the tool, and what you need will come to you from the invisible reality. Remember: You are free. You are now coming to that recognition.

How To Confront Self-Doubt

Self-doubt began in the Garden of Eden, when the serpent whispered in Eve's ear, prompting her to doubt her relationship to the One Mind and Its voice, which we call the "first" voice. When the serpent spoke to Eve, it introduced a second voice, thereby challenging the first voice that had guided her until then. The word "doubt" means "two." Doubt is the second voice, which, when attended to, paralyzes action, freezes our sense of self-confidence, and creates a stoppage of movement in our physiological system.

This exercise may help you overcome self-doubt.

The Serpent's Curse Exercise

Close your eyes and breathe out three times slowly. Know you are doing The Serpent's Curse Exercise to make yourself confident and that it takes a few seconds.

Wearing whatever you need to protect yourself, see the serpent of doubt snaking toward you and trying to hypnotize you into doubting. Look away from his eyes, grab him by the tail, and send him snaking away from you as you curse the one who has come to curse you. Breathe out one time and see yourself refusing to eat the apple as the snake disappears. Know doubt has been conquered for now.

Breathe out and open your eyes.

Self-doubt has many sources and many degrees of intensity. No one exercise can be equally useful to everyone but *The Serpent's Curse* is quite powerful.

A man came to see me after suffering several severe traumatic experiences. He had functioned extremely well before he had these experiences, but now doubted himself in many ways, doubted that he could ever overcome the damaging effects of the traumas.

I asked him to describe the image of doubt. He saw a black hole. I asked him to correct this image, while knowing that as he did so, the doubt was disappearing. He saw himself closing up the black hole by sewing it together with golden thread. He experienced a great sense of relief.

I recommended that he correct the black hole every time he experienced doubt.

He reported soon after that while the doubt still made itself felt, it was less and less perceptible, like an ache that was fading away.

This powerful exercise is easy to do. Imagine your self-doubt, then *correct* it. Whatever you see is the correct image for you. However you correct it is the appropriate correction for you. Just remember: this is imagination, the language of freedom, a God-given potential in each of us, and, as I stated earlier, anything is possible.

How To Confront Indecisiveness

Indecisiveness is much more than carefully considering your options. Some of us are quick to make decisions; some of us are slow. But sometimes we simply cannot make a decision, no matter how much consideration we give it. We are paralyzed, stuck. If you have trouble making a particular decision or find yourself in a state of general indecisiveness, use the next exercise to free yourself to decide.

The Mummy's Wrappings Excercise

Close your eyes and breathe out three times slowly. Know you are doing The Mummy's Wrappings Exercise to rid yourself of indecisiveness and that it takes 15 to 20 seconds.

See yourself between two mirrors. In the left mirror, see and feel yourself to be a mummy, experiencing all the feelings of being a mummy. Catch the end of the bandage lying over the navel and unwrap it. Make the bandage into a ball, and throw the ball into the center of a large, dark cloud that has formed in the blue sky above you. See the cloud breaking up, releasing its stored rain, washing over you, and cleansing you. Breathe out one time.

In the right mirror, see yourself singing, dancing, and happy. Then wipe that image away to the right with your right hand. See the mirrors disappear, breathe out, and open your eyes.

How to Confront Disquieting Feelings

We each of us live in a sea of feelings. We like that person but don't like this one (who, unfortunately, may be our boss). We enjoy doing this but not that. We are comfortable with small groups, nervous in large groups. We become angry when people make jokes about minorities. We feel agitated when we go to work, relieved when we return home. The list does not end. Happily, most negative feelings pass (even if they regularly reappear); they do not enshroud us. But some disquieting feelings overwhelm us – feelings of loss, of fear, of hopelessness.

Wiping the Mirror Clean Exercise

Close your eyes and begin your even, regular breathing. Then breathe out three times slowly, counting backwards from three to one, each exhalation being a new number. Know you are doing the Wiping the Mirror Clean Exercise to free yourself of disquieting feelings and that it takes 15 to 20 seconds.

At one, you breathe out again and see the one become a zero. See the zero growing a bit in size and becoming a circular mirror. Looking into the mirror see and resolve any lacks or limitations you sense in yourself. Each time, see the particular lack or limitation, breathe out once, and wipe the image away imaginally to the **left** with your **left** hand. Now, in the blank mirror, see and resolve repression and frustration; then envy and acquisitiveness; then insecurity and uncertainty; then doubt and hesitation; then hostility. Wipe the image away to the **left** each time.

When you finish, turn the mirror around to its other face and see yourself tall, smiling, bright, and healthy.

In this exercise, you can see and resolve any feeling that is upsetting you. See the feeling in the mirror. After resolving it by image, wipe the new image away to the **right** with your **right** hand.

After you finish, breathe out, and open your eyes.

In this last exercise in particular, we are seeking to free ourselves of conditioned, childish responses and allow ourselves to become adults. Becoming adult is a spiritual act. It is not really a mystery, though it is not always easy. It is also a stepping-stone to illumination and self-realization. Adult means to grow up. Sounds simple, yet it is difficult to execute for most people.

There is not enough space here to examine adulthood from the kabbalistic perspective, but I would be remiss if I left the subject without identifying five of the main ingredients to permit attainment of adulthood:

- Bearing loss

- Sacrifice

- Turning hate into love

- Following the ten laws of balance – or, as they are more commonly known, the Ten Commandments

- Taking the Three Vows for inner growth:

obedience (the willingness to obey
the invisible reality)

chastity (faithfulness to the One)
and

poverty (giving up the need to
acquire excess material wealth in
favor of the wealth of Spirit that
comes from the invisible reality)[2]

[2] See my descrition of the three vows in *Healing Into Immortality*, pp. 86-87.

Chapter 8.

SURVEYING OUR BODY'S HEALTH

In the previous several chapters, our focus has mostly been on mental and emotional matters such as anxiety, worry about money, and being thrown off balance. In the next few chapters, we turn to another large area of everyday concern: physical health.

In the practice of Visionary Kabbalah, health and healing is a holy focus, for it is a province of God, as God says in the 15th chapter of Exodus, "I Am the healer." We need to understand this literally: "I Am the healer." To maintain a personal relationship with the divine healer, we strive toward achieving, maintaining and acting in balance; another term for this is moderation. Once we put ourselves under the wing of the divine healer, we are provided, in return, with the grace bestowed by the universe, an influx of beneficence, and a sense of self-restoration.

When we look at the modern medical establishment, we hardly see moderation and balance. We see a system inundated with sufferers, and a system whose costs are skyrocketing. Why? Because "I Am the healer" is entirely ignored. There is no place for Spirit in this system, which puts its emphasis almost totally on the cause-and-effect understanding of health and illness. Cause is seen as a material source which, when corrected, brings about health, defined as cure. If this belief is the truth about health and illness, why has it not made a dent in the health mania and the disease enveloping the country?

However, when we direct our gaze toward the invisible reality and utilize its possibilities, we can use the practice of imagery to take charge of our health in a new, more beneficial way.

One of the most important things we can do for ourselves is survey the state of our health. The medical establishment says tests of this or that are the true measure of whether or not something is out of balance in our bodies. I do not denigrate the findings of medical science – though I believe they have their limits – but I strongly assert that since we are born of Spirit and have a relationship to the divine, we can be our own best assessors of our health. We do not need to wait until a symptom expresses itself or until we go to a doctor for a checkup to determine the condition of our physical health. Through mental imagery, we can scan our health in a few seconds, any time we want. We are, in effect, doing our own mental MRI!

You may recall the example of the woman who correctly saw in an imagery exercise that one of her fallopian tubes was crusted over. There are many such examples. Here is one more. A woman was scheduled to have an operation for fibroids. The gynecological surgeon said he could not determine exactly how many fibroids there were. The woman did an imagery exercise where she entered her body. She found the uterus, explored it, and determined how many fibroids existed. When the operation was performed, the number she discovered turned out to be correct.

You can come to such awareness for yourself. Just as you seek self-mastery in the mental and emotional areas, so it is your challenge to attempt self-mastery, to the degree that it is possible, in the area of health.

How to Monitor Your Health

In this brief chapter, we focus on two imagery exercises you can use to scan and evaluate the state of your health.

The Lake of Health

Close your eyes. Breathe out three times slowly. Know you are checking the state of your health and that it is taking up to 10 seconds.

See yourself high up in the Andes at a lake that is eight thousand feet above sea level. Tell the lake that you want to know the state of your health, and that you want the lake to reveal to you your outer and inner body. Then look into the crystal-clear, quiet water and see yourself inside and out. Breathe out and open your eyes.

If you are healthy, you characteristically will see either a golden color or pure pink, blue, or green. If you are ill, you will see a gray, black, or bluish pink at the site of the disturbance.

The Field of Health

Close your eyes. Breathe out three times slowly. Know you are scanning your health for up to 10 to 15 seconds.

See yourself as a general outside your tent at the head of the field of your body. Your bugler is next to you. You have a large golden flag blowing in the breeze at the top of your tent. At all important points on the field of your body are other tents with flags flying and buglers stationed next to them. Have your bugler blow his bugle and hear each bugler at each tent answer in turn. See the flags blowing at the same time and see their colors. Breathe out and open your eyes.

If any sound is discordant or a flag does not blow or shows a black or gray color, some change is taking place that bespeaks a disturbance or illness.

Now, if you uncover a disturbance, its nature might be clear enough to try to resolve the problem on your own by using imagery exercises or other techniques you have found useful. In the next chapter, we explore the use of mental imagery to resolve physical problems.

You might alternatively choose to deal with a disturbance by finding the appropriate health practitioner to remedy the situation. That is up to you. You may recall that both of the women who employed mental imagery to discover their gynecological problems ultimately used gynecological surgeons to remedy them.

Chapter 9.

DEALING WITH PHYSICAL AILMENTS: INFLAMMATION AND MUSCLE SPASMS

In our kabbalistic understanding, we believe that ailments do not arise out of the blue or, for that matter, from germs that have randomly located themselves in our bodies. They arise in the social/moral milieu in which we participate, and it is by examining this milieu that we identify the significance of an illness and the meaning it contains. As you will see, in the kabbalistic approach to illness, we do not ask "why" a person becomes ill with this or that ailment. We look for the situation/experience/event in a person's life that is mirrored analogically in the ailment. More of this later.

For the space of this chapter, I am going to bypass the essential question of context. I want instead to underscore the basic principle you use to devise mental imagery for problems of physical health and to show you as simply as I can how to apply mental imagery to alleviate physical ailments. Then, once you understand the basic principle, you will be able to become a more active participant in your own healing by taking greater charge of your health in a responsible way, and thereby advancing in the self-mastery that Kabbalah seeks for every person. Whether your physical ailments are chronic or acute, however deeply embedded they may be, you will have the means to use mental imagery to bring yourself relief, though, in many cases, not full understanding.

In effect, this chapter is step one in a two-step process. Only in the next chapter do we examine step two, which takes us beyond the symptoms and experiences of physical ailments to their sources.

Here, to show you the nuts and bolts of devising and applying mental imagery, I consider two physical ailments that frequently arise in everyday life – inflammation and muscle spasms.

How to Create Mental Imagery for Physical Ailments

The basic principle in devising imagery to help relieve physical ailments can be stated in four words: Go to the opposite. Why the opposite? You may already know the answer: because our natural state is to be in balance. When we suffer from an ailment, physical or emotional, we are pulled out of balance. We need to restore our balance and we do this by *going to the opposite.*

Let us see how this might be done with inflammation.

If you have an inflammation – any sort of inflammation anywhere on or in your body – what do you need to do to find its opposite? You begin by asking questions about the characteristics of inflammation. For example, what is the color of inflammation? The name tells you. When you have an inflammation, you are inflamed, on fire; you are red. And how do you neutralize red and bring yourself back into balance? Blue neutralizes red, so you use blue.

But how do you neutralize your red inflammation with the color blue? Look again at the meaning of inflammation – inflamed, on fire. You need to put out the fire. What better way to put out a fire than with blue water?

Dig a little deeper. What provides a really forceful dose of blue water? Though you might see something else, the object that occurred to me in formulating this exercise was a fireman's hose. The image of a fireman's hose is especially appealing to me because the jets of water come out so forcefully in the form of a spiral, and a spiral is a cleansing movement in our bodies. Spirals fill our lives. Our hair grows in spirals; an embryo as it becomes a fetus grows in a spiraled movement, and it is known that the movement of growth in the created world has the form of a spiral.

To remove the flame, we use the spiral movement of blue water gushing forth in a pressurized counter-clockwise spiral stream.

Now we are ready to apply the image.

The Fireman's Hose Exercise

Close your eyes and breathe out three times slowly. Know you are doing The Fireman's Hose Exercise to remove inflammation, and it is taking you 5 to 10 seconds.

Walk outside your front door, and you see a fire hose attached to a hydrant in the ground. Lift the hose and direct a counter-clockwise blue spiral jet of water onto an inflamed area to see it cleaned out and the flame disappearing. Return through your front door with the inflammation gone. Breathe out again and open your eyes.

If you have an inflammation, do this exercise three times a day, up to 21 days.

Now let us apply the principle of going to the opposite to create an imagery exercise for removing a muscle spasm.

The Muscle Expansion Exercise

Let us suppose you have a cramp in your legs. You can start the process of finding an opposite by asking yourself: what is a cramp? The answer that comes to you may be along the lines that when a person has a leg cramp, it seems as though the muscle is in spasm. If cramp leads you to spasm, you then might ask: what is a spasm? You may not exactly know. If not, you can look it up in the dictionary. You will see there that a spasm is a contraction. You might now observe to yourself, my muscles are in a contracted state and because they stay contracted, I experience a cramp.

So now you ask: What is the opposite of contraction? "Yes, I see," you might say, "expansion." Okay, now what would you do to create an expansion in your contracted muscles? What sort of opposite would bring expansion to your contracted muscles? You probably would like to stretch these muscles. Of course, you can physically stretch the muscles, but remember, this is imagination, where anything can happen.

How would you like to stretch your muscles, then, in your imagination? I can tell you what I did when I had a cramp. In my imagery, I put my hands *inside* my leg, and I stretched the cramped muscles, teasing out the knots and elongating them. I separated the knotted strands from each other and made them long and glistening white, so they came back to a gleaming state, a natural state. And I saw that where I had the cramp, my leg became very long because with the muscle contraction, my leg also had contracted.

I have extended my leg; I have extended the muscles; and I made the muscles very long, to act in opposition to the spasm.

Of course, I begin the actual exercise sitting in the Pharaoh's Posture, breathing out and in three times, and telling myself that I am doing *The Muscle Expansion Exercise* to relieve the spasm, and it is taking me 15 to 20 seconds.

If you have need to try this exercise, see what happens to your cramp and the place it occurs after you apply your image. You can re-do the exercise any time if the cramping comes back. With the principle of going to the opposite, you can work on any physical ailment.

Some of you may find that it is not so easy at first to determine an opposite. Just keep asking yourself questions, as we did when looking for the opposite of inflammation and muscle spasm. Feel free to use the dictionary to explore synonyms. If one question does not bring you answers, other questions will. Keep probing. The opposites will appear.

The more often you do this, the more profoundly you will see that you have at your disposal a powerful tool to help you become your own healer, aligned with the divine healer.

It is time now to move to step two, which asks such questions as: How does it happen that my skin is inflamed? How does it happen that I have a cramp in my leg? In the phrase "how does it happen," I am being slightly roundabout because I do not want to use the word "why." In Kabbalah, an ailment encapsulates something that has gone out of balance in a person's life. Determining this significance is the subject of the next chapter.

Chapter 10.

IDENTIFYING AN AILMENT'S SOURCE

As we have observed, Visionary Kabbalah contends that good health goes along with observing the laws of balance, otherwise known as the laws of spiritual life. Health is an expression of living in balance and harmony in our relationship to spiritual powers and forces that are greater than us and that want to collaborate with us. When an imbalance arises within our social/moral matrix – when one or another part of our lives goes beyond a tipping point – it will also be experienced in our physical system.

Spiritual healthcare is not a matter of determining cause-and-effect relationships. It is quite different. It is a matter of relating part to whole, out of which comes a revelatory discovery of the entirety.

Here is an example from personal experience, which at first seemed only a casual encounter. I had had a difficult time parking my car in front of my office. I had to maneuver into a tight space, with an SUV behind and a sedan in front. The sedan's driver was sitting in the car.

As I was leaving my car, the driver of the sedan stepped out to apologize for not moving her car forward to make things easier for me. She explained that her battery was dead and that she was waiting for AAA to come and help her.

I often speak up in situations where perhaps others would not. I asked her how she was experiencing her inner battery.

A startled look crossed her face, but she understood my point at once.

103

"You think there is a relationship between the car's battery and *my* battery?"

I responded that nothing happens by chance, so there had to be a relationship.

She said that, as a matter of fact, she had felt tired, drained, and run down in the past week. Her chronic asthmatic state had worsened, and she was on her way to see her doctor when the car battery went dead.

I was happy to reply that she indeed had seen her doctor – me – and I left for a moment to retrieve a paper in my office on using mental imagery to treat asthma, the very condition from which she was suffering. I had written the paper several years earlier with a number of colleagues (Dr. Elizabeth Barrett, most notably). I said she might find something useful in it and wished her well.

I never heard from the woman, but for me the incident is an example of the kabbalist principles that nothing happens by chance and the universe is always sending us what we need. You may say that it is only random chance that the woman in the car in front of me was suffering from asthma and that I once happened to have been involved in writing a paper on how to use mental imagery to relieve it. But think about it: Is such an explanation any more credible than my belief – confirmed again and again in many areas of my life and work – that there is order in the universe?

More immediately, the incident also shows how revelatory experience is applied to healthcare, leading to discoveries that enlarge a sufferer's understanding of what is disturbing his or her well-being. One aspect of revelatory experience is to discover relationships between things that are seemingly unrelated. In this instance, we were able to see the relationship– called analogy – between the outer battery of the auto and the inner battery of the rundown woman.

Whether or not you are comfortable with the part-to-whole relationship I see in this encounter, I think you will be able to see that a comparable part-to-whole relationship exists with an ailment and its context. For instance: heart ailment – disappointment in a love relationship; liver ailment - unresolved anger; lung ailment – internal crying that is held in and not expressed; gall bladder ailment - chronic envy or jealousy.

Identifying the Source

To examine the part-to-whole relationship so that it reveals the context, let us keep with the example of leg spasm. Let us say that you have resolved a leg spasm using the kind of imagery we discussed in the previous chapter. Let's say as well that you are still not satisfied. You want to know "why" you had a leg spasm. This means, in the kabbalistic approach to illness, you want to know the relationship of the leg spasm to some other aspect of your life. Specifically, what is the analogy of this ailment to some other spasm or contraction in your life? Here we come to the heart of the matter. The "why" has given way to the analogical "what." What is happening in your life that the ailment portrays? What is the message of the ailment?

To discover the source of a physical ailment such as a leg spasm – a form of contraction – you will find it useful to extend the notion of contraction into your life. You can ask yourself: "What has contracted in my everyday life that has reflected itself in physical contraction?" A bit more technically, you might say: "What function does the spasm in the leg serve? And of all places for it to happen, it's in the leg? What function does the leg serve?"

Let your mind scan what is happening in your life right now to see if there is anything that makes you upset or unhappy. Maybe it is something that happens regularly. Or maybe it is more like a single sharp incident. Most often, it reflects some relationship difficulty, though the link is not always a direct one.

A specific experience might immediately spring to mind. You might say: "Well, you know, I was so angry at my boss today that I wanted to kick him. Of course, I had to hold back, because I could have wound up without a job. I just wished I could have done it."

Now, you kick with a leg and you had a leg cramp, but how does your desire to kick your boss reflect as a leg cramp? It happens as a result of two opposing pulls. The desire to kick your boss is a pull in one direction; your refusal to act on your desire is a pull in the other direction. There is now a mental-emotional- physical link created in our mindbody world. When we are caught between two pulls, the habitual response is to move in a third way, creating a symptom. The symptom represents the torque or the resultant tension between two pulls. It is an expression of a wish (to kick the boss) plus a fear (that I will be fired if I do). It represents an opposition in ourselves. You wanted to initiate a kick, but you resisted and stopped yourself from doing it. By stopping, you prevented a movement of your leg. The result in this case is a muscle spasm.

A symptom like a leg cramp is the body speaking in its own language. The function of earthly human existence is to communicate. We are social-dwelling creatures who live in communication with each other, always communicating to ourselves or others in one way or another.

Our emotions are part of this communication; they speak. We feel happy; we feel joyful; we feel angry; we feel sad; we feel depressed; we feel gloomy; we feel morose. We are always feeling and speaking. Our mental life, speaking to us all the time, is also part of the communication within which we live. It is saying things like: "I'm pondering this, I'm contemplating that, I'm obsessing about this, I'm in doubt about that, I'm feeling elated." The mental life is always speaking; the body is always speaking.

So, what you are doing when you examine the source of an ailment is learning to read its message by going back to see how it connects to the sources of imbalance. Once you discover these sources, the ailment's message becomes much clearer. Moreover, the awareness of the message, in and of itself, gives you a direction for healing.

As you can see, this is all fairly simple and easy. It takes some practice and some persistence, but it is a tool that all of us can master. And as simple as it seems, it is never less than illuminating, for it can widen our lives in powerful ways, opening us to the invisible reality that is at the heart of the kabbalistic perspective and that always gives us what we need.

The Woman with a Leg Cramp

A woman came to see me because she wanted to know how to deal with a persistent and painful leg cramp.

We began by exploring its source. The woman quickly realized that it was connected to a conflict she was experiencing with regard to her husband. He was out of work, and from her perspective he was not striving hard enough. She wanted to stir him into becoming more active in the family's survival. She wanted to kick her husband in the behind because he was not providing for the family. At the same time, she did *not* want to kick him because she felt loving toward him and thought this would be an unloving act.

Additionally, she felt afraid to kick him. So the woman felt anger and love towards her husband, as well as some fear.

"What's the fear about?" I asked.

"Well, if he doesn't provide enough income, we're not going to be able to live adequately. We may not have enough food on the table. We may not be able to survive. We have a new child. We have to live, and I'm afraid we won't have enough food."

I stopped her from going further.

"I'm sorry, but you're talking about something that I can't really respond to. I feel for your situation, but you're talking about the future, and you're talking about a goal. You're talking about some possible outcome that may or may not happen, and we can't talk about outcomes. We can't talk about goals because they are fixed images, idolatrous thoughts. They are future-oriented, and the future doesn't belong to us. The future belongs to the divine healer." For us it is an illusory region.

She was puzzled. She was a spiritual person and accepted that the future belonged to God, but she could not see why I viewed her fears about her family's future as idolatrous.

My kabbalistic explanation went roughly as follows: The healer is the invisible reality. If we put ourselves in the place of the invisible reality, trying to force people -- in this case, her husband – to satisfy our need for the goal we want, then we have usurped the knowledge and power of the invisible universe, and we have made ourselves the great God. And when we take over the role of being the Almighty in this presumptuous way, we prevent the invisible reality from entering into our experience and providing us with whatever we need. We break the covenant and contract made between Abraham and God: that if we accept and devote ourselves to the invisible reality, the invisible reality will give us everything that we need.

At the same time, when her mood is determined by what another person – in this case, her husband – says, does, thinks, or feels, she, paradoxically, is making herself into a slave, not into God.

I told the woman that all distressing feelings are attached to thoughts about either the future or the past, and that both the future and the past are illusions: the first because it does not exist, the second because it is dead, gone, and buried. Feelings of shame, guilt, and regret are attached to thoughts about the past. In her case, her feeling of fear was attached to thoughts about the future, inducing in her a conditioned habitual pattern of behavior that is common to the miseducation we all receive in this society. She was following the accepted pattern of feeling, acting, and then thinking. Her feeling of fear prompted her to take an action that carried with it some unpleasant thoughts about her husband.

However, in becoming mature in our relation to experience and living in the world, we want to reverse the pattern of feel-act-think to think-act-feel.

The idea that she might approach her situation in a new way excited her.

What she needed to do, I explained, was a twofold process – an inner process and an outer process in the world. The inner process came first.

I explained that seeing is one form of think-ing and that mental imagery, then, represents a form of thought. Given her spiritual inclinations, I added that mental imagery is also a prayer given form. We might call it a way of thinking with/to God.

We then set the conditions for her to begin the work. I told her to sit straight up in the chair, her arms on the chair arms, feet flat on the floor. She was to close her eyes, breathe out and in three times slowly while setting her intention inwardly to *reverse* the debilitating conditions and situation that affected her relationship to her husband.

I asked her to think/see the situation as she would like it to be. She said, "I see my husband working. I see my husband going to work – getting into the car, and driving away to work."

"How do you feel?"

She said, "I feel a sense of peace. I haven't really experienced something like this for such a long time with my husband because it's been such a really diffi-cult time economically, and it's had such an unhappy effect on our relationship. I just feel a sense of peace."

Now she needed to move to the second phase of the process – the outer phase.

"What I'd like you to do now in your home life is consciously think about his going to work and having a job, and then *acting* as if he has the job. Pretend, if you like, that he is working, and behave toward him as if he is working. And then see what feeling comes to you when you respond to your situation in this new way."

In this twofold process, we reverse the usual feeling-acting-thinking pattern into a thinking-acting-feeling pattern. Through mental imagery, the woman is internally thinking. Then in her outward life she externalizes this inner thinking and consciously thinks that her husband has a job and is going to work. She then acts by behaving as if the thought is a current reality, and she explores the feeling that accompanies this behavior.

What happened a short time later was no surprise to me, since it commonly happens in my practice. The woman called me with the good news: "I wanted to let you know that my husband just got a job."

"You see," I said, "you let the universe in. You allowed the universe to operate with you and to cooperate with you."

She said something like, "Everything has worked out so well, I just want to thank you." From my perspective, I deserved no thanks. The aid came from the invisible reality to which she had opened herself. She began by wanting to know why she had a painful leg cramp that would not go away. Using mental imagery to identify the situation that was expressed in her leg and then using other practices – especially reversing the usual practice of feeling-acting-thinking – to apply her new knowledge, she found a new way to be in the world and in her inner life.

For the sake of emphasis, let me say this another way. While imagery initiated the dynamic process that took place, imagery alone did not lead to the change that occurred. The woman had to apply the knowledge that came to her through imagery. She had to apply it inwardly and outwardly. And then, having done that, which meant living in a new way, she could do no more. She was not God. Whatever else that was to happen had to come from a force greater than she. And, in her case, it did.

Chapter 11.

COMBATTING INNER TERRORISTS: THE KABBALAH OF ACTION

Any book that intends to take a reader through a typical day, showing how imagery can help a person meet common challenges, has to talk about what we call inner terrorists, for they often are our daily companions. Any book that puts imagery within the profound context of Kabbalah needs also to talk about inner terrorists, for the high aim of Visionary Kabbalah is to show us the way to freedom, while the demonic aim of inner terrorists is to put us into bondage and kill us.

For most everyone on earth, the state of existence is bondage. The bondage can be literal – as it is for an incredible number of people on earth today – or can be of one's own making, that is, an enslavement that is experienced emotionally, mentally and through the patterned experiences of one's social environment. This form of bondage is the work of the inner terrorists, analogous to outer terrorists, against whom we must battle as vigorously. Inner terrorists are inner entities, mental children, or inner demons formed by our attitudes, feelings, beliefs. They are waging a guerilla war against us, day after day, their sole purpose being that we succumb to death.

Our inner terrorists take root early in life. They have their beginnings in the miseducation, false beliefs, and conditioning that our family, our schooling, and influential others unknowingly and unintentionally foist on us and perpetuate. Not only beliefs but whole patterns of conditioning are instilled in us in our early years, when we have little self-awareness so we cannot see that we are being put on a path where we regularly create inner terrorists.

In the ancient Western esoteric wisdom, in which Kabbalah plays a prominent part, inner terrorists were called *egregores* – the ancient Latin term for any artificially created inner demons. *We* create these artificial demons – Pinocchios that lie, for example – in the guise of thought forms. In effect, they become our mental children. As soon as they appear, they need attention, nurturing, and feeding; and, like many children do with their parents, they often end up controlling us.

In this chapter, we examine how we create these inner terrorists and how, through will and imagery, we can free ourselves from them.

How We Create Our Inner Terrorists

How do we create our inner terrorists? When we feel anxious, when we feel worried, when we feel scared, we are really creating an artificial demon. These feelings are always attached to false beliefs, which like seeds or weeds planted in consciousness, take root inwardly and grow into these entities or *egregores*. Once we create these demons, they have a continuing effect on and influence over us. With this new understanding, we can now combat these demons through the use of will and imagery, the two root practices of the kabbalistic path.

An Inner Terrorist At Work

A good example of how someone creates an inner terrorist is the experience of a woman who came to see me. She viewed herself as eminently fair and a person of impeccable integrity, but she often had been taken advantage of or cheated.

As we began discussing this apparent paradox, she quickly discovered that when she was young, she in fact did take advantage of her friends. When this happened, her mother severely admonished her. At the time, the woman vowed *never* to cheat again, and she had made every effort to reject and deny this quality as a genuine, authentic potential in herself.

What her vow and her effort amounted to was to create an inner terrorist. By denying her cheating tendency, she gave it breath and life inside her. As if it were a shadow, it "followed" her everywhere.

Now that the woman's secret belief was out in the open, accepted and *owned*, it could be *dis*owned. That is, she could now freely choose to carry out the possibility or not. The shadow was now seen in the light of day. As soon as this happened, the cheating incidents virtually disappeared from her life. The denial of her authenticity gave way to the only real control we have in life, to take charge of our beliefs. She understood it is as valid to be a cheater as it is to be honest when looked at in an unbiased, unprejudicial way. This is true for all characteristics in human life; all choices are genuine. And, all have their consequences.

What the Inner Terrorists Want

Our inner terrorists want to keep us enslaved; they want to maintain the status quo; they do not want us to succeed; they do not want us to become free; they want us to remain afraid, anxious and conflicted. Their central avowed aim is our demise.

Our task throughout life is to free ourselves from the enslavement we bring upon ourselves through our creating and nurturing our inner terrorists. We free ourselves by constantly watching and recognizing how these inner terrorists have intruded into our life space. They are the weeds choking the garden of reality we have been given at birth to maintain.

How To Recognize Inner Terrorists

How do you recognize an inner terrorist? What are the signs that tell you that an inner terrorist is operating? *Any* emotional state you experience as distressing – no matter what the name – is the sign of an inner terrorist. Your grammar also contains signs that an inner terrorist is present. When you speak in the future tense about what "could, would or should happen", either in your own inner dialogue or to somebody else, an inner terrorist is operating. If you are talking to somebody in the past tense about "should have, could have, would have", an inner terrorist is operating.

When you are feeling pain – whether emotional, mental, and/or physical – it is a sign that an imbalance exists, and in any condition in life where you are feeling an imbalance, a terrorist is operating.

When you make a fixed goal, an inner terrorist is operating. When you become worried about results and outcomes, a terrorist is operating. The terrorists operate in many tricky ways.

Even when you are comforting yourself, a terrorist may be operating. For example, when you try to convince yourself to change your ways, a terrorist is operating. "Oh, I shouldn't do that," you might say to yourself. "I really shouldn't. Come on, now, you're not acting the right way. Yes, I'm going to try and do it differently." Once you start talking to yourself this way, trying to convince yourself about how you *should* act, how you really need to change things, how you have to be more alert, more aware, etc., etc., etc., it is a sign of inner terrorism. All such ostensible self-improvement talk may seem a healthy form of giving yourself some internal support, but you are really under the sway of a terrorist. Like a motivational speaker, he or she is subtly – or not so subtly – offering a standard you are urged to meet. Invariably, you will fail to meet that standard or, instead of becoming the person you want to be, you will focus your energy on not being the person you do not want to be. So, if you are the kind of person who keeps admonishing yourself not to do this or that any longer, you would do well to stop, because you are really supporting a saboteur in your midst.

Clearly, our job is to be on constant watch as guardians of ourselves, and to take active steps to rid ourselves of the terrorists. Otherwise, the terrorists will get rid of us. We keep on the job and on the alert all the time.

How to Confront the Inner Terrorists

Here are two main tools for dealing with the inner terrorists, which we also term false selves. The first is an active awareness; the second is mental imagery.

Active awareness is an act of will. As soon as your awareness tells you that an inner terrorist is operating, you can inform your higher Self. The higher Self is a kind of master inner guide. It is a not-easily definable endless stream/pool/well of limitless awareness that always tells us the correct way to address our needs. Once you inform the higher Self that there is an inner terrorist, the higher Self will give you the correct order to get rid of it – for example, "Stop feeling anxious" or "Drink a cup of tea." Just the act of awareness in itself, before the higher Self is called upon, can eliminate the false self. Each time a false self appears, you deal with it in the same way.

Once you take charge of your inner terrorists and start to remove them from consciousness, your true Self becomes increasingly awakened, and begins operating much more actively as the observing function of your higher Self. The awareness function now comes into prominence, and as you remove the inner terrorists, you create a space of freedom for something new to come in. You will also find that you experience a sense of lightness, of greater peacefulness. If you are anxious, the anxiety will likely disappear. You will feel calmer. These are all steps to your healing, your freedom, and your turn to the invisible reality.

However, if you do not make a space, you remain enslaved by the terrorists, who block the way for anything new. You remain stuck and slowly decay.

Mental imagery, the second major way to confront and conquer inner terrorists, is no different than the imagery you have been practicing throughout this book. It is the imagery you use to change your life – emotionally, physically, spiritually. Here you focus on the destructive forces within you that you have created. To wipe out your inner terrorists, you are on an eternally vigilant "search and destroy" mission.

Here are two exercises you can use to eradicate your inner terrorists to improve your well-being and open space for the many possibilities of the new.

The Flushing Exercise *(devised by Dr. Peter Reznik)*

Close your eyes and breathe out three times slowly. Know you are doing The Flushing Exercise to get rid of the inner terrorists, and it is taking up to 15 seconds.

Spontaneously, see one of your inner terrorists in front of you. See what he or she looks like. Or perhaps it is a creature. And above this terrorist is a water trough. You pull the chain, the trough door opens and the water torrentially comes pouring over this inner terrorist, flushing him or her or whatever the creature might be, down the drain. And as this terrorist disappears down the drain, know that this being is going to the center of the earth where it will be completely incinerated by fire. Sense and feel what happens, and then breathe out and open your eyes.

The Key to the Prison Door Exercise

Because our inner terrorists enslave us, the aim of this second exercise is to end the enslavement. There are many ways to stop our enslaved relationship to life. As you become more skilled in the ways of mental imagery, you probably will find your own approach. But, I think you will find this one useful.

Close your eyes and breathe out three times slowly. Know you are doing The Key to the Prison Door Exercise to free yourself from enslavement by your inner terrorists, and it is taking 15 to 20 seconds.

See yourself in a prison cell. Have a light with you if you need one. You can have any kind of light you wish since anything is possible in the imagination. Then look around the cell and discover the key that unlocks the door.

When you find the key, unlock the door to let yourself out of the prison. Keep the key with you, knowing that you can return to the cell any time you need or wish to. Outside the prison cell door find the staircase that ascends. When you find the staircase, climb up the steps to the door that you find at the top of the steps. Open the door and find yourself coming out into a clear, bright, light open space. Know that you have taken the step toward ending your enslaved mentality. And after finishing, breathe out and open your eyes.

I would like you to look at two particular aspects of this exercise. First, notice that I said to keep the key with you so that you can come back to the cell if you need it. Even though, as Kabbalah makes clear, our real aim in life – our real wish and desire – is to become free, oftentimes freedom scares us. It is characteristic of a number of people with whom I have worked, that when the door of freedom has opened, and they see the light beyond the door, they immediately pull the door shut. They do not want to take the step into the clear open space.

Some people make it known that they want to hold onto their illness; they want to hold onto their familiar lives. Not seeking freedom or, after finding it, turning one's back on it and rejecting it, is to be acknowledged and honored as a respectable approach to life. It is a genuine choice, your choice. You keep your key to make that choice.

The second thing to notice, for some of you at least, is that when you came out of the prison cell, you may have met a guard or some officer there. It is very common in imagery exercises to find guardians or keepers of certain places – keepers of the door, keepers of the space you want to enter, from whom you must ask permission to do so.

If you meet such a guardian, ask if you have permission to enter the room or space that the guardian is watching over. If the guard says yes, you give your thanks, and continue on your way. In some cases, the officer will ask you for something in exchange for permission to go on. If this happens, find something on your person to give the guard as a payment for continuing.

If the guard does not give you permission, this is a diagnostic sign for you. It shows that to some degree, you may be rejecting your own freedom or may be resistant to it. You may not be ready for the change(s) that can ensue. You can try again, to see if resistance is still operative. If so, don't fight it for now. Return to waking life, breathe out, and open your eyes.

Try again tomorrow.

With persistence, you will "overcome" – in the word of the civil rights anthem – and move into the space of freedom, beginning to live the life that Kabbalah offers to us as a possibility for fulfillment in this passage on earth.

You may need to do these exercises again and again. As I said before, we are masters at creating inner terrorists; they are masters at finding ever new ways to insert themselves into our lives and thoughts. Be vigilant; seek self-awareness; employ mental imagery.

Chapter 12.

HEALING THE PAST

For many of us, disturbing memories from the past are frequent unwelcome visitors to our daily lives. These past experiences influence our behavior and our feelings about ourselves. We suddenly yell at one of our children and hear the voice of our father coming out of us. We speak sharply to a salesclerk because her lack of attention reminds us of our mother. In such episodes, we feel trapped in the past. We stop being who we want to be, and we revert, unknowingly and, it seems, helplessly, to former versions of ourselves that we thought we had "out-grown." We wonder: Can we ever put an end to the continuing presence of the past? Can we ever out-grow it?

Kabbalah says yes. Directly contrary to the prevalent view of experience – that it makes us who we are – Kabbalah allows us to understand that the personal past content of life experience has *no* true relevance to our current presence in the now of this moment. What is genuine about the past, as it pertains to where we find ourselves today, is the conditioned patterns/habits that were established and that keep being played out in our current life experience. From the perspective of Kabbalah, then, our primary concern regarding the past is with "the then in the now" – the beliefs from earliest life that continue to operate in the present.

There are various ways that the past can keep us from moving forward in our lives. Some of us have painful memories that we are unable to forget. Some of us keep remembering events, perhaps painful traumas, which we cannot let go of, even though we want to. Some of us have pasts that seem like the albatross hanging from the neck of the ancient mariner. Perhaps most common are the troubling false beliefs that have dogged us since our earliest life – the "old wine" that continues to pollute "the new bottle."

Again, mental imagery is the tool to self-mastery and achieving freedom. The painful and disabling connections to the past that shackle us can be corrected by the visionary process of imagery. This frees us to get on with our lives in a new, fulfilling, perhaps creative way.

How to Heal the Past

The past can intervene in our present lives in different ways. Here I describe a variety of exercises with different emphases. Choose the one that is most applicable to you. You can use any of these exercises to put the past to rest as an unsettling influence in your life.

The Correcting the Memories Exercise

Some of us find that there are certain situations in our lives that keep coming up and that we keep referring back to. These are our painful memories – ideas or remembrances of the past that are still playing a role in our lives. We do not seek these memories. Instead, they seem to be there always, waiting to fill us with their pain.

Painful memories operate in us as a conditioned response. When something occurs that reminds us of a painful past event, we experience a pain similar to the pain we experienced before. To free ourselves of the effect of painful memories, we need to correct them so that we are no longer locked in a conditioned stimulus-response cycle.

A research study conducted in New York City is a good example of how a conditioned stimulus-response works. The subjects were a group of about 35 former heroin addicts who had lived in Harlem when they were addicts. They now lived outside of the city, had been freed of their heroin addiction through the use of methadone, and, at the time of the study, were also freed of their methadone addiction. With the permission of the former addicts, a researcher bused them back to the sites of their drug days. They drove over the George Washington Bridge, came down the West Side Highway, got off at 125th Street in Harlem, and were taken to the street corner where they used to buy their drugs. As soon as they saw the street corner, which functioned as a stimulus, they all went into withdrawal – the conditioned response to that stimulus. Put another way, the former addicts responded to the memories of the past as if the events of the past were taking place in the present.

All that is needed to evoke a conditioned response established by past events is a stimulus that reminds you of a previous situation. Then you respond as you felt in the past. Any cue, any molecule of a cue, will elicit a previous response. That is what happens to us when we experience painful memories, and why we invoke mental pain so often. Some current experience – it could be the way someone lifts a hand, an inflection that someone uses in speaking – elicits the response associated with the previous experience, and we respond exactly as we did in the past.

In a conditioned experience, a stimulus comes and a habitual response follows – stimulus, then response; stimulus, then response; stimulus, then response – as if the experience were as fixed as flipping a switch (the stimulus) and a light turning on (the response). This happens, in effect, by itself, without our consent.

The truth is, when we see something that we know, what we usually see is our memory of it rather than its actuality. For example, when you wake up in the morning and open your eyes, you are not seeing your bedroom as you originally saw it. You are seeing your memory of the room. The memory of things is always the experience that is going on in your recall of your life events. When you meet someone you know on the street, you are not meeting the person anew; you are starting with a memory of the person. Similarly, when we recall something from our lives, we recall the memory of it – something other than the actual thing.

I had a vivid experience of this in a high school course in journalism. One day while we were all sitting in the class a fight broke out suddenly, unexpectedly and seemingly spontaneously. After the fight ended, the teacher explained that she had arranged it, and she asked all of us to write a report of the experience. There were 25 people in the class, and every person's report was different.

What happened in the journalism class is a common phenomenon. The point is simple: Memories are often variable; they are malleable and do not exactly recreate the original event. Memories are not the facts; they are our vision of the facts. So there is always some shift that can be made in memory.

In every stimulus-response arc, there is always a space of freedom. Even in the quickest biological stimulus-response arc that we know of, there is 1/250th of a second of freedom. So it is in our lives; there is always a space of freedom, and everywhere we can, we want to make a space of freedom for ourselves.

What happens if you insert a new response into your memory of the past? When the stimulus comes in your current life, instead of activating the habitual response button, it activates the new memory, which now acts as the buffer between the stimulus and the habitual response. When the stimulus hits the buffer, you no longer get the habitual response. You get a brand new one, and the new response ignites in you a new attitude, a new possibility, a new option, a new avenue of approach, a new habit.

The imagery exercise of *Correcting the Memories* is a way of replacing an old memory with a new one, thereby undoing the conditioned, seemingly fixed link between the stimulus and response of a past experience.

In this exercise, we locate the past memory (or memories) that continues to bring us pain. The experience of a young man, who came to me because he had become increasingly concerned about not having spoken to his mother for ten years, illustrates this process.

He was constantly angry with her, he said, so angry that for a decade he had not communicated with her. I asked him if he could give me an example of his anger. In particular, was there a memory in his life that he could point to that would exemplify his whole range of experiences with his mother that would precipitate the feeling of anger. I explained to him that a single memory can contain and stand for an entire roster of memories that point to a recurring situation in one's life or to a persistent feeling or attitude.

Something came to him immediately.

"I remember when I was a little boy," he related. "I was five years old, and she took me to a department store. She was buying something, and I got bored and started to run around. I was running here and there, and I was kind of making a commotion. My mother was so embarrassed by what I did that she grabbed me by the ear and pulled me out of the store. I saw everybody laughing at me, and I was furious with her. That would be an example of how I feel about her and her treatment of me."

"Could you go back and change the memory?" I asked.

"What do you mean, change the memory?"

"Make something new happen. Change your attitude in front of the event. Do whatever you want to correct this situation that happened."

Surprised and a little puzzled, he agreed. Sitting in the Pharaoh's Posture, he closes his eyes, breathes out three times slowly, and goes back in his imagination to the department store. He sees himself there as the little boy. He sees his mother take his ear – because it helps to face the pain for a moment to make the correction - and as she's pulling him out of the store, he sees himself taking her hand off his ear, putting his little hand in her big hand, and sees both of them walking out of the store hand-in-hand. The people, instead of laughing at him, are smiling at them. He looks up at his mother, she looks down at him, and they are smiling at each other.

After the session he went home, called his mother, and spoke to her for the first time in ten years, reestablishing their relationship.

When you correct a memory, you are not changing the *fact* of what happened to you. What happened to you happened to you. What you are correcting is your *recall* of the fact. You are *correcting* your memory, the memory of the fact. Your memory can change, and when you change it, you are changing the link between stimulus and response. Create a new memory, create a new response.

This process of altering our memories is a very significant facet of our ability to bring about healing. Once we put the past in its proper place, it no longer unnecessarily occupies a space in our consciousness. The space becomes uncluttered to allow a new creation to enter. The term "creation" here is tantamount to healing – that is, coming into greater order and complexity.

The Burying the Past Exercise

Sometimes there is a piece of the past that you are unable to relinquish. Even though you know it is past and want to let it go, it still restrains you from moving ahead in your life. People have frequently come to see me because they want to let go of a prior relationship that broke up, but find they cannot. As a result, they cannot establish a new relationship, although eager to do so. So we do the *Burying the Past Exercise.*

Close your eyes and breathe out three times slowly. Know that you are doing the Burying the Past Exercise to let go of the past, and it is taking up to 60 seconds.

You see yourself walking along a country path. The path is cluttered with rocks, which you clear to make the path passable. At the end of the path, you find a tree. You sit by the tree, and from the ground around you, you pick up a leaf. Using sap on the leaf as ink, you write on the leaf all that you can recollect that has pained you from your past - the regrets, the obstacles that inhibit you from going forward.

Now indicate when you want the past to disintegrate by writing a date on the leaf. Then dig a hole and place the leaf in the hole, knowing that you are burying both the leaf and the past, which like the leaf, is still somewhat alive but will eventually disintegrate. Fill the hole with dirt, and after finishing, quickly go back to the path that you followed to the tree, seeing if anything is different on the path as you return to your starting point.

When you reach the starting point, you breathe out and open your eyes, knowing that your past is buried.

On the way back from burying the past, you may note something special along the path. You may find it different from the rock-cluttered path that you originally started with. If this happens, as it does for many people, the changed path is a confirmation that the exercise has had an effect.

Some people do not see any changes. This sameness is a diagnostic showing that there is still an intention or a tendency to hold onto the past. How the path looks will give you an indication of your progress in regard to fulfilling your intention to bury the past.

If you do not see anything different about the path on the return trip, simply continue doing the exercise for a period of up to 21 days. At some point, you are likely to see some change, confirming that the exercise has taken root. When that occurs, you needn't continue the exercise. The job is done.

Retracing the Past Exercise

Some people want to change their relationship to whole swaths of their past, sometimes even to their entirety. In spiritual life, certainly, the past is to be regarded as over, done, ended, dead, and buried. Only the now has significance and meaning. The two-part exercise called *Retracing the Past,* an unusually long exercise, may help you change your relationship to your past.

You do this exercise knowing that you are doing a two-part exercise called *the Retracing the Past Exercise* to create your past anew and that it is taking up to seven minutes for each part.

Part 1

Close your eyes and breathe out three times slowly.

(1)   Looking into a mirror imaginally, see, sense, feel, and live the significant disturbing places and events of your life. Begin from the earliest time in your life that you can remember, perhaps from the earliest infancy you can recall, and move in sequential chronological order up to the present moment. You do not have to recall all of the significant disturbing places and events of your past. The specific places and events you recall are representative of similar themes. Remember, old wine in new bottles.

(2)   After finishing, you breathe out one time slowly, and looking into the mirror, you see yourself now going back in time, seeing the significant places and events of your life in **reverse** sequential order – from the immediate moment back to the beginning. As you go back, you are correcting all of these disturbing events and places by changing your memory of them. For those that you cannot correct this way, see yourself washing them out of the mirror to the left with a giant fireman's hose. To wash away or to move an image to the left is to place it in the past that no longer exists.

(3)   After finding you have turned these experiences around, you breathe out one time slowly, and in the mirror, see, sense, feel, and live these new corrected events and places in chronological order, from earliest life into the present moment.

You are now living a different past and a new now.

(4) Then you breathe out one time, and in the mirror, see how you have to live these new corrections in a year, two years, and five years from now. Then, when you are ready, breathe out and open your eyes.

Part II

In the second part of this exercise, done right after the first, you now focus on **inner** aspects of your life from the past. To do this, close your eyes and breathe out slowly three times.

(1) In the mirror you again see, sense, feel, and live the disturbing faults and errors of your life, the significant ones, starting from the earliest childhood or infancy experiences that you can recollect and moving in chronological order up to and through the present moment. Remember, these are the significant faults and errors of your life, each one representing a whole group of a particular sort of fault or error.

(2) When reaching the present moment, you breathe out one time slowly, and in the mirror, see, sense, feel, and live yourself correcting these faults and errors, going in reverse chronological order from the present moment back to and through the earliest childhood or infancy experi-

ences that you can recollect. For the faults and errors that you are not capable of correcting, find yourself washing them out of the mirror to the left with a giant fireman's hose.

(3)   After having reversed these experiences, breathe out slowly one more time, and in the mirror see, sense, feel, and live these new corrected faults and errors in chronological order, from earliest life up to the present moment, sequentially living with a different past and a new now.

(4) Having completed this correction, breathe out one time again and, with these new corrections in place, see how you have to live them in one year, two years, and five years from now. After finishing, breathe out and open your eyes.

Changing and correcting much or all of one's past with this exercise requires assiduousness. When doing it, I recommend that you do it every morning for 21 days. Always remember to give yourself the name of the exercise. Say, "I'm *Retracing the Past* with the intention of correcting my life. And it's taking me up to seven minutes for each part."

Now, in any of these exercises, if you find that you don't seem to be making any headway, don't fret, because change is often a matter of continuous practice. You will see progress within 21 days. Keep up your determination to do the work, your investment in the work, and your willingness to commit to your self-healing and health. Keep looking to see what the experience gives you, what the images say to you. This will provide you with a gauge of how you are progressing.

The exercises to change your relationship to the past, like all the exercises in this book, are designed to allow you to break from your conditional and conditioned life. Unlike behaviorism, kabbalistic practice endeavors to help you create a new value system where you may discover the worth and validity of invisible reality and the presence of forces associated with that reality – in sum: spiritual life.

Chapter 13.

SLEEP TIGHT: IMAGERY EXERCISES TO BRING SLEEP

We come to the end of the day.

The Kabbalah of Light is still operative in sleep. Sleep has a restorative function, allowing us to recharge our batteries and keep us in rhythm, the rhythm of the active daytime and the restful night-time. Sleep is also the occasion of the visions of night called dreams, which can be read and explored with a spiritual understanding. Here, however, in keeping with the book's day-in-the-life theme, we focus on the recharging aspect of sleep through preservation of sleep, including help falling sleep.

Although sleep is the natural needed end to a day, sometimes it does not come easily. Difficulty in falling asleep represents the intrusion of daytime concerns and activities into the quiet and calm that is necessary when going to sleep. As we know, day and night are clearly divided from each other. It is unnatural when the dividing line is crossed, and the line needs to be restored.

Closing the Door on the Day

If you have trouble going to sleep, I recommend the following exercise. Use your imagination to bring anything you need to close the door on the day which is intruding into the night, and to build a barrier between the time of sun and the time of moon, between light and dark.

137

This worked well with a friend. He was a statistician in a government agency and was compiling a large body of data that would help determine whether certain departments that were concerned with assisting people below the poverty level should or should not have their budgets increased. Politically speaking, he had a liberal perspective, and for that reason he was all the more determined that he be unaffected by his bias.

Always something of a perfectionist and a worrier, and so something of a poor sleeper, his intensified effort to be accurate and objective preyed on his mind when he went to bed. Only after much tossing and turning could he fall asleep.

I suggested that he use the Closing-of-the-Door-on-the-Day Exercise, which he tried.

While lying in bed with his eyes closed, in his imagination he gathered all the papers that he was studying and the computer on which he was writing his report, together with his notes about the material he still needed to obtain and examine, and put them into a large safe that he saw in his office. There, he also put several superiors from the office and one data collector whose work always needed to be redone. When he firmly closed the door to his office he found himself in the dark, unburdened, and quickly drifted into sleep.

He continued to use the exercise while he worked on finishing the report to his satisfaction, a process that took several weeks. He slept soundly during this time, and in the morning always woke up feeling fresh and energetic.

Here is another exercise to separate the thoughts of the day from nighttime sleep.

Flowers in the River (*devised by Sheryl Rosenberg*).

While lying in bed with your eyes closed (no special breathing needed), see yourself lying by the bank of a swiftly flowing river. You are surrounded by flowers. Smell their fragrance. Pick one. Take each preoccupying thought you have, place it in a flower, put the flower in the river, and see and hear the flower being carried away quickly downstream, disappearing as it is carried around a bend to the left in the river.

Continue this exercise until you fall asleep.

Interrupted Sleep

At times you fall asleep easily, then suddenly you are wide awake, tense and full of thoughts about daily concerns. This occurs frequently with some people. If it happens to you, try this exercise to restore your sleep.

The Sandman Exercise

While lying in bed, close your eyes and breathe out seven times slowly. Take your daily concerns and leave them in a metal box at the edge of the sea. A giant wave comes to shore and takes the box into the ocean, where it sinks to the bottom.

Breathe out one time. Now, lie down on the sand. As you look out to the horizon, see the sun setting below the horizon. Close your eyes while lying there, and know and sense that the Sandman approaches you and sprinkles the sand of sleep over your closed eyes, putting you back to sleep. Keep your eyes closed and sleep tight.

Children and the Dark

Sometimes, especially in children, there is a fear of the dark and a concomitant difficulty in falling asleep. This difficulty usually disappears when the child turns nine or ten years old. If it continues, I would recommend an imagery exercise in which the child sees himself or herself surrounded by a golden dome of light encasing the whole body, protecting the child from any and all danger. The child now sees him/herself sleeping peacefully.

There is no need for the child to name the exercise, but it is helpful to point out that this exercise can help him/her fall asleep safely.

Chapter 14.

AWAKENING TO SPIRIT

In the remaining three chapters, I want to go beyond the morning-to-night framework of the previous chapters to examine three basic spiritual issues that apply to the whole of our lives. In this chapter, I examine how we consciously can move toward Spirit. In the next chapter, I examine spiritual freedom. In the concluding chapter, I speak about the nature of the invisible universe, the canopy under which we all live.

It often happens that going through your day with the awareness that comes from practicing mental imagery, an interest in matters that are beyond your usual concerns in the day-to-day material existence spontaneously awakens. You have glimpsed the presence of the invisible, immaterial universe and the way it can help you live your life in a more peaceful, contented, conflict-free manner. You may also have seen that in opening yourself to what the invisible reality has to offer, there is a promise of long-lasting health, happiness, and well-being.

In its simplest form, awakening to spirit means getting up every day and beginning it with an imaginal experience, which brings you into the day with a new attitude toward the day about to unfold, and perhaps, with a new perception about yourself and the world you are meeting.

Both this chapter and the next one are intended to further your movement on the path toward the spiritual life envisioned in Kabbalah, whose whole purpose might be summarized in a simple but profound motto: *"To bring life to life."*

Bringing Life to Life

My practice is replete with examples of suffering people who come to my office experiencing their life situations and conditions as a curse. But they leave knowing the curse is really a blessing: the blessing contained in making the turn toward Spirit. Spirit is inherent in our birth but laid dormant by faulty conditioning. It is re-ignited by the alchemical process of turning the lead of destructive habits into the gold of personal transformation.

There are four exercises in this chapter, each of which speaks to a different aspect of moving closer to Spirit. The first deals with giving up destructive habits and becoming a freer person, the second with knowing your moral nature, the third with awakening to Spirit, and the last with claiming your spirit by joining the divine Spirit. Any and all of these exercises can be done each day as often as you think them necessary.

There are times when some people want to break free of their injurious habits and put themselves in touch with a source of truth. They want to become considerate, contributing, harmless people. They want to repent - to think in a new way - and connect with the invisible reality. If you are experiencing such a moment in your life, I recommend the *Turning from Our Errors Exercise,* an exercise that involves repentance.

I perhaps should explain that repentance, simply put, is the capacity to turn away from our harmful habits and conditioning and make corrections for those errors. In kabbalistic understanding, the broad perspective of life is that we make errors and we are given the opportunity to correct them. Thus, it is

said in the mystical tradition of the West that forgiveness and mercy *preceded* the creation of the
world. Without the possibility of forgiveness and
mercy, we would all perish very quickly. But God
knew that errors were forthcoming and, so, gave us
repentance to enable us to live.

Turning from Our Errors Exercise

Close your eyes and breathe out three
times slowly. Know you are doing the
Turning from Our Errors Exercise to repair
your injurious habits and to connect with
the invisible reality, and it is taking 30 seconds.

Breathe out one time. Know, live, and
feel repentance as a universal phenomenon.

Breathe out one time. Know that
repentance is the highest expression of
man's capacity to choose freely.

Breathe out three times. Sense and
feel the relationship of repentance to time.

Breathe out one time. See experience
changing time's significance from future to
present.

Breathe out one time. See and know
how by turning again, we are able to truly
repent.

Breathe out one time. See and know
how, by turning from our errors, we are
truly repenting.

Breathe out one time. See, know, and
feel how repentance brings an answer only
when we really turn from our errors.

Breathe out slowly, and open your eyes.

The Ten Commandments Exercise *(from the Old Testament)*

(1) Don't Put Any God Between You & God;
(2) Don't Create/Erect Idols, Nor Make Graven Images;
(3) Don't Take God's Name In Vain;
(4) Remember And Observe The Sabbath;
(5) Honor Your Father And Mother;
(6) Don't Murder;
(7) Don't Commit Adultery (Mixing);
(8) Don't Steal;
(9) Don't Bear False Witness;
(10) Don't Covet

This is a long exercise. Read it over a few times before you begin. You will see that its ten parts mirror the Ten Commandments listed above. You can do all of it or just the portions – the commandments – that seem especially relevant to you. Over time, you may discover that portions you passed over have become relevant. By doing these exercises, you can personally experience the deep meaning of the Ten Commandments – otherwise known as the Ten Laws of Truth, the Ten Precepts, or, as I noted earlier, the Ten Laws of Balance. Laws mean that which has perpetuity over a long expanse of time, as from generation to generation or millennium to millennium. Commandment means the call to action concerning an immediate situation or circumstance facing you in the moment.

Close your eyes and breathe out three times slowly. Know that you are doing The Ten Commandments Exercise to know your moral nature and it may take thirty seconds to three minutes.

(1) Know and feel that there is no other god but God. Breathe out three times slowly.

(2) Imagine yourself in the museum of your past personal life. See yourself breaking all the statues you have placed there and ripping up all the paintings that you have made. Breathe out three times slowly.

(3) Become a seed planted in the earth. Sense and know your growing as this seed, and know from where the nutrients come. Breathe out three times slowly.

(4) See and live yourself walking backward through the day. Note what you experience. Breathe out three times slowly.

(5) See, feel, and know that your parents are your creation. Be reborn in a new way. Breathe out three times slowly.

(6) See and feel anger. Take one step back from it, look at it again, and laugh. Breathe out one time slowly. Choose life. Be aware of what you are feeling. Breathe out three times slowly.

(7) Know how to separate the oil from the water. Do not let them get mixed again. Breathe out one time slowly. See and know that when we let them get

mixed, we adulterate our own life force. Breathe out three times slowly.

(8) See and know what is meant by the statement, "To steal from others is to rob yourself of life. To steal from yourself is to rob others of your presence." Breathe out three times slowly.

(9) See, sense, and know that silence is golden. Breathe out one time slowly. See this silence becoming golden. Breathe out one time slowly. See this golden silence encircling you. Become aware of what you experience. Breathe out three times slowly.

(10) See yourself sitting at a sumptuous banquet table. You are with complete strangers. Breathe out one time slowly. Eat your meal, but begin each course by giving away your portion to one of the strangers. Note what you feel. Breathe out one time slowly, and open your eyes.

The Rising with the Sun Exercise

This is an exercise, as I said, about waking to Spirit.

Close your eyes and breathe out three times slowly. Know you are doing the Rising with the Sun Exercise to waken to Spirit, and it takes 60 seconds.

You are in a long narrow ancient Egyptian barque on the water in a dark tunnel. It is so dark that you can discern absolutely nothing. You hear the water around you lapping about the boat and the tunnel walls and the oars in the water.

Then, at the front of the boat you can begin to see the dim outline of a sail. It can barely be made out. You go to the front of the boat and find the sail that can be made out more clearly flapping in the breeze. At the bottom of the sail, you find a ball that can be seen more clearly as more light begins to enter.

As the scene becomes clearer and clearer, you see that the ball is a golden one and that its light brightens all, and that the sail, attached to the mast, is a radiant and transparent one. Your body becomes the mast and is covered by this radiant transparent sail as you watch the sun rise very slowly in front of you. You find yourself, as you watch the sun rising, beginning to rise with the sun. You then remove the sail from the mast by lowering it, and then putting it around your shoulders as a white cape. Become aware of the sensations that happen and continue watching the sun rise.

Descend from the boat and come back in your imagination to the chair in which you are sitting, physically opening your eyes and continuing to watch the sun rising, and describe the sensations to yourself.

Some time ago, I worked with a middle-aged woman who was very successful in her field of public health. She was Jewish, but having been raised by non-practicing parents, she had lived her life as an agnostic. She was married to a fellow agnostic, and they had two children. The family celebrated something they called Hanumas, but the household was entirely secular.

Then, during the AIDS outbreak, the woman witnessed the deaths and suffering of many people whom she had come to know through her position in public health. A large number of these people were middle class, as was she. Some were religious, some were atheists, some were spiritual. All the latter believed in something beyond the material and saw a meaning in life that was larger than the visible world. This was also true of many of those who were committed to a particular religion.

She saw no clear difference in the suffering of people whether they did or did not believe in a particular religion, were or were not religious, or did or did not have spiritual beliefs. But she experienced an internal change. She told me that watching the painful, sometimes agonizing deaths around her, she came to feel that she no longer could trust the material world. She did not know how else to say it: she had lost trust in the world.

Her husband was understanding and sympathetic. She agreed with him that she was reacting to the onslaught of the seemingly meaningless and unceasing deaths she had been witnessing. She understood that as time went on, she might find a way to accommodate herself to this experience and to regain her trust in the world. But for now, she felt unmoored. She felt full of sorrow and tears - whether for the dead and the dying or for herself, she did not know. Walking to work, she often did not know where she was going. She had to stop, take a deep breath, and remember where and who she was - a middle-aged woman walking to her job in public health.

She had heard of me from some of the people with whom she had come into contact and knew that I had, as she called it, a spiritual orientation. Since she no longer had trust in the world, she wanted to know if my spiritual orientation might help relieve her distress. I said it was possible. After further discussion, I suggested that I lead her through *The Rising with the Sun exercise.*

At the end, I asked her to describe her sensations. Speaking slowly and softly, she said she felt lighter and less agitated. She wasn't sure, she said, but she thought she felt more peaceful, almost as if she were being supported.

I recommended that she do the exercise three times a day for twenty-one days and to call then, or anytime sooner, if she felt the need to do so. I did not hear from her until the end of the twenty-one days. She reported that she continued to feel stronger and peaceful and that the feeling of support had grown. Most importantly, she said, she no longer dreaded going to her office. She felt recommitted to her work, no matter how painful the experiences it brought to her.

The next year she began taking classes with me on the Kabbalah of Light.

Joining the Divine Exercise

This is a very short, very profound exercise.

Close your eyes and breathe out three times slowly. Know you are doing the Joining the Divine Exercise to claim your

150

spirit nature, and it takes a few seconds.

See your body become half a circle.
See the other half as the Divine. See,
sense, and feel what happens. Breathe out
and open your eyes.

Do this exercise each morning for as long as you like.

Chapter 15.

FINDING SPIRITUAL FREEDOM

Kabbalah, as I have said, is a guide to freedom, spiritual freedom. What does Kabbalah mean by freedom? It means finding our own self-authority, independent of outer or inner suggestions and repetitive habits; and overcoming the inevitable enslavement created by conditioning that dominates our lives. As human beings, we are *all* subject to conditioning imposed by earthly life. Conditioning engenders faulty habit patterns that eventually lead to our wearing out, becoming ill, decaying and dying. In the practice of Kabbalah, then, to be spiritually free is to be an unconditioned being.

According to Kabbalah, there are four unconditional processes that make up the freely acting/living being we are all destined to become. These are:

- unconditional thought, expressed through intuition;
- unconditional feeling, expressed through love;
- unconditional action, expressed through faith;
- unconditional language, expressed through imagery.

I believe that the practice of mental imagery enhances the other three processes. (I shall have more to say about these processes in the concluding chapter.)

Throughout this book, we have regularly touched on becoming free of particular destructive

151

situations, expressed in false beliefs, physical symptoms or harmful habits. It has been a constant (not always explicit) theme of our work. Here, as we come toward the end of this exploration, I want to offer three concise exercises through which we directly move ourselves to spiritual freedom. These exercises are brief – in one case almost nonexistent, it is so quick. They may seem as insubstantial as feathers, yet they take us to the heart of Kabbalah and to the heart of our deepest endeavor as human beings.

In one of these exercises, the imagery is to see the present as no time. I once gave this exercise to a mathematician whose work was well beyond me. I thought the exercise would appeal to him. One reason he became a mathematician, he told me, was because numbers were so free. He originally came to me for a physical problem. Sometime after the problem was resolved, he returned to ask me why he could not feel as free as a number.

When I told him to close his eyes and see, sense, and live the present moment as no time, he began to smile. Then a look of surprise swept over his face. Then happiness. "Ahhhh," he said, dragging out the sound. "That's what the present is."

I do not know what he saw, or whether he saw what only a mathematician could see. But I believe that whatever he saw was an expression of spiritual freedom.

To translate his experience into words would have seriously diluted his experiential moment.

The Exercises

Each of the following exercises is done in the morning. The third exercise, you will see, has three parts. You can use any part, any combination of parts or all three parts. The exercise you choose to do and the part or parts of the third exercise you choose to do, is your decision. Let your intuition – your unconditional thought – guide you.

Three Freedom Exercises

(1) Close your eyes and breathe out three times slowly. Know that you are doing an exercise to bring you to spiritual freedom and that it is taking a few seconds.

Live and know why freedom cannot be connected directly to our physical relationship to life. Breathe out and open your eyes.

(2) Close your eyes and breathe out three times slowly. Know that you are doing an exercise to bring you to spiritual freedom and that it is taking a few seconds.

See, feel, and sense how freedom cannot happen without being in a physical body. Breathe out and open your eyes.

If you do all three parts of the following exercise one after the other, you keep your eyes closed throughout. The second part of the exercise, of course, is the exercise I gave the mathematician who wanted to feel as free as a number.

(3) Close your eyes and breathe out three times slowly. Know you are doing an exercise to bring you to spiritual freedom and it is taking a few seconds.

Regard yourself as a shining flame burning brightly without name and form. Know and see how the complete meeting with the infinite is eternally within ourselves. Feel free! Breathe out and open your eyes.

Close your eyes. Breathe out three times slowly. Know you are doing an exercise to bring you to spiritual freedom and that it is taking a few seconds.

See, sense, and live the present moment as no time. Breathe out and open your eyes.

Close your eyes. Breathe out three times slowly. Know you are doing an exercise to bring you to spiritual freedom and that it is taking a few seconds.

Sense and feel how the imagery process allows us to live the presence of the Present. Breathe out and open your eyes.

Chapter 16.

N THE INVISIBLE UNIVERSE

is exploration by pulling together the ~~central strands~~ of kabbalistic practice I have touched on throughout this book. The aim of our practice is to open to Spirit so it may flow through us. In finding true freedom, we take a leap into uncertainty.

As a jumping off point, recall the story of the woman who had a leg cramp. She wanted to kick her unemployed husband to find a job but, out of love and a fear that he would leave, did not kick him. In one way the woman wanted to be God – she wanted to control her husband. In another way, she made herself a slave, because she came to believe that her happiness and comfort depended on what her husband did. Through our work together, the woman did what was necessary to give up her desire for control and end her enslavement. She then proceeded to align herself with the invisible universe.

Each of us can do what this woman did in aligning ourselves to the universe. The essence of the process is to reverse the belief that you "must" control the outcome. Instead, making a new choice in life, you cede control to the invisible universe, the divine healer. You do this by taking the step we call *faith* into the darkness of the invisible.

I want to explore this choice of faith because it shows how the practice of mental imagery in the spiritual context of the kabbalistic perspective brings us independence. Faith replaces the tyranny of our conditioning with freedom, a true inner power, and is the microcosmic equivalent of the macrocosmic power of the Almighty.

The State of Being Dependent

Faith has many components. One is aligning yourself to the moment of now and allowing the invisible reality - which operates in, and only in, the now - to make its way to you and to give you what you need.

Faith was very far from the thoughts of the woman with the leg cramp. We must ask: Why did the woman try to play God, prodding, provoking, stimulating and pushing her husband into doing what she wanted for herself? To reach a non-disturbed state, to experience pleasure and avoid pain – which is exactly how our archetypal progenitors, Eve and Adam, went awry. They were fooled into thinking they needed more than the paradise they already had, and they were duped into believing they could substitute themselves for God and become God. The woman wanted to be in the non-disturbed state and was depending on her husband to give it to her. She believed that if he did what she wanted she would feel pleasure, and that as long as he did not, she would feel pain. And this is when she became a slave, allowing her mood to be determined by what her husband would or would not do. In her attempt to become God, she became a slave. She became a dependent soul, dependent on the external world to fulfill her need. And to the extent that we are dependent on the external world to fulfill our needs, we all become slaves. We become dependent and conditioned.

We condition ourselves to be happy only when others do for us what we think we need. Conditioning means always being dependent on something else to give us worth, merit, value, authenticity, however you want to phrase it. And as we do this, we therefore can never find in ourselves the worth, merit, value, authenticity that we want. It always has to come from somewhere outside of us.

The moment the woman stopped attempting to manipulate and control the outcome of her husband's actions, she created a new space - a space to allow the universe to come to help her. The universe cannot come to help us unless there is a space for it in which to operate: "the space of freedom." And once we allow this space of freedom to open up - in the case of the woman, by separating herself from the goal and from the result - the universe will always come to fill it in to our benefit (even if, at times, we do not recognize it as such).

The State of Being Unconditioned

In opening ourselves to the invisible reality, we are changing from being conditioned beings to becoming unconditioned beings. How do unconditioned beings live?

For example, what would be unconditional feeling? Love. I love you, and I do not need anything back from you to make my love meaningful or to give it worth. It is what it is. I do not necessarily need to be loved in return, because *love is.* It is an unconditional state. That is true love.

What is unconditional action? Faith. The willingness to leap into uncertainty, the willingness to make up your mind and choose, or decide without indecision or doubt. Without recourse to what the world thinks, you come to trust yourself and your relationship to invisible reality.

What is unconditional language? Image. The image comes from an invisible source. It is the sacred language. Through image we come to the storehouse consciousness where images repose. We plunge into this storehouse consciousness to find the images, and the process is not dependent or contingent on anything around us. Images stand on their own, unassociated with any other content.

What is unconditional thinking? Intuition. Intuition is unconditional thought because it is not dependent on the outside; it is dependent only on listening to one's inner voice. It is not influenced by the external world, where we are suggestible and capable of being influenced virtually all of the time. But if we ask questions of ourselves - as we have done in the exercises in this book - and hear the answers come to us, then our intuition is functioning. When you are listening to the inner voice that comes to you, the language of truth channels itself through you. You are now thinking unconditionally and independent of the world.

The Space of Freedom

If you doubt the universe's direct role in your life, learn through your own experimentation: create a space of freedom by renouncing outcomes and results, and discover if the universe comes to fill it up to your benefit.

The act of permitting the space to open up is entirely in each person's hands. We are all born with free will and choice to fulfill in our own lives the covenant made between Abraham and the Universal One Mind long ago. We are showing our devotion, appreciation, openness, and love toward the invisible reality by allowing it to enter into our lives. It is an act of love to allow the invisible world into our lives.

Why do we block the invisible reality from helping us? We do it unwittingly. The faulty beliefs induced by our institutions and by the educational systems in which we are involved block us from finding our own way to fulfillment, balance, health, and realization. Instead, we become goal-oriented, result-oriented, outcome-oriented: we *materialize* our aims. Rather than seeking God's presence in the material world and the overall value of the invisible world, we seek interest in what manifests itself in the experiential world, treating our material world as the endpoint beyond which there is nothing more.

The more we want to materialize our lives, the more concerned we become with the realization of goals. Materialization involves goal making. This leads us into a closed system: Goals mean materialization and materialization means goals. It is a finite system, and by the Newtonian laws of physics, every finite system has to decay. But, rather than simply being our material body casing, we truly are open systems, where there is no decay because there are no fixed images. We set our intentions and allow the invisible reality to communicate with us. By not allowing ourselves to live as open systems, we block our own possibilities and the fulfillment of our human potential. Is this how, deep in our hearts, we want to live? Wouldn't we rather live so that we become fully ourselves, drawing on the universal practices that allow us to work to balance ourselves and maintain our health and general well-being as we advance with confidence into the uncertainty that fills our lives on earth?

Faith is the key here, for once we give up the delusion of control, we give ourselves and the results of our efforts over to a higher power. While we open the door to healing through our active participation, it is not ours to demand that we heal. Whether or not we heal is a matter between each of us and our Creator. At the same time, we live in peace with the result, for we understand that is in our best interest; it is what we need at that moment and at every moment.

In the practical "occidentation"[3] that is the basis for this book, the practice of Kabbalah encourages faith, hope, and caring for oneself in a health-giving, meaningful, enriching way. Faith means there is a way out of bondage; hope shows the way out; caring means to live by universal law and love. It is my fervent prayer that you become imbued with faith, hope, law, and love, on your road to freedom and liberation.

[3] I coin this term to emphasize the Western basis that informs the book. "Orientation" means the Orient, whose doctrine of Spirit differs markedly from our Western approach.

APPENDIX

NOTES ON HOW-TO CREATE
YOUR OWN IMAGERY

To help you on your way, on the journey this book recommends, I want briefly to review the process of devising your own imagery, which you likely will want to do as you proceed.

We already have seen that a basic technique of creating your imagery is to go to the opposite. In some instances, you may discover, the opposites emerge spontaneously.

A student connected flames with the emotion of anger. I asked him to sit in the midst of the flames, letting them flare up around him. At first, he was somewhat frightened, but eventually he entered into the flames (probably because he trusted me and, therefore, trusted himself) wearing a suit of asbestos. As he sat in their midst, he saw their heat taken up by the clouds above him. The clouds became laden with water, burst open, and doused the flames with rain.

With this downpour, his anger abruptly stopped. Such experiences are commonplace in my practice. The imagery had brought forth the opposite of the flames.

You will see that as you become your own imagery authority, you will gain a greater trust in yourself, a greater faith in yourself, a greater awareness of yourself. And as you practice finding the images that you know are best for you, coming as they do from your inner life, your intuition will consequently grow and grow and grow. Intuition – unconditional thinking – is a way to become connected to your inside truth. You will be hearing an inside voice, accessing an inside voice, and receiving an inside answer that comes through to you. The practice of mental imagery is one of the great practices for reaching and developing the capacity of your intuition.

The Pictures in Words

A key to imagery is that every word that we use – every noun, every adjective, every adverb – has an image associated with it. This does not mean that the particular image of any one of us is universal - that the image you have for a particular noun or a particular adjective is the same as the image I have. Not at all. From person to person, images may be quite different. But the basic principle holds. Each of us always associates each word with an image.

The procedure for accessing this image is simple. Ask yourself what image is associated with this or that word. The answer will come.

This is a general principle, a process of healing that is given to us. If you ask yourself questions, answers will come to you. *But you must ask.* Answers are available to us only if we ask. The ancient Western spiritual tradition says, "Ask and you shall be answered; seek and you shall find; knock and the door will be opened to you." So it is a matter of asking, and when you do, you will hear, feel or sense an answer. It will come to you immediately. When somebody once asked me, "How would you look being peaceful?" what immediately came to my mind was lying in a hammock which was swinging very gently back and forth stretched between two trees. This is not the image that may come to your mind. But I'm sure if you ask for an image for calm or peaceful, the image appears instantly. Let it happen as easily as that for anything else you are working on.

Let us practice discovering the word images each of has by looking at the state of being we identify with the word "angry." In this book, we have not done much with anger, though for many it is a distressing and painful feeling. How can imagery help us deal with anger?

Close your eyes. Breathe out slowly three times, knowing that you want to deal with anger..

Ask yourself: What is the image of anger? Let the image come spontaneously. You do not have to edit it. Just allow it to emerge. There are no rules of logic in this situation, so anything can come. It does not have to make "sense."

Many of you likely had a spontaneous image. For those who did, breathe out one time slowly. Go back into that image and now correct it - reverse it, change it, transform it. See, sense, and feel what happens. And after doing so, breathe out and open your eyes.

The purpose of the exercise is to gain mastery over the feeling rather than allow it to be your master. Feelings are never destroyed. Rather, they are transformed. In the case of anger, by transforming it, we become harmless to ourselves or others.

What we did to picture anger, you can do with any word. What is the image of love? What is the image of fear? What is the image of confidence? What is the image of Spirit? What is the image of failure? What is the image of progress? What is the image of ability? What is the image of father? What is the image of space? All of us have all the answers, as different as they might be.

Using Imagery to Defuse Distressing Feelings

People today often talk about *managing* distressing feelings, as in anger management, for example. But why manage when you can transform? Imagery allows us to change the energy of distressing feelings by transforming it for constructive purposes.

One person who imaged anger saw it as shattered glass. When I asked her to correct the image, she picked up all the pieces and created a glass sculpture. You can see in this example – an excellent illustration of going to the opposite – that a creative and transformative act took place.

We need to understand that a creative force is embedded in anger, and when the force is channeled constructively in a new direction , the energy is likewise redirected from being destructive into being constructive. When you begin to handle distressing feelings through imagery, the very same energy that was used negatively is used positively, freeing yourself of distress and increasing your ability to create.

Perhaps the best-known and most familiar examples come from the lives of visual artists. One is Vincent van Gogh. For whatever reasons, perhaps epilepsy, van Gogh experienced bouts of anger. And you see how it became transformed into his wondrous paintings! Anger sparks creativity. Beethoven is another example of an artist who redirected anger, transforming it into his great musical works. In our time, Jackson

Pollock would throw his anger at the canvas, through the medium of paint, to form his abstract images.

All these artists used the energy of their anger to create something beautiful. Using imagery in our own ways, we can do the same with our anger and other distressing feelings. All feelings are useful - including the feelings that cause us distress - if they are transformed.

Many of us reflexively suppress distressing feelings. It follows from the false belief that the purpose of living is to reach a non-disturbed state to have pleasure and avoid pain. Thus, when the painful emotion comes, we want to suppress it, so we run from the feeling, try to push it under the rug or deny it. We turn to drugs, alcohol or other intoxicants to gain a "non-disturbed" state.

Any disturbing feeling state needs to be faced, not suppressed. By facing the feeling in its image form, we gain a sense of our own power to take charge of the feeling by a simple inner process that changes the field. We then have a new perception and conception of our situation and can choose to actively involve ourselves in creating change.

In addition to anger, the long list of familiar distressing feelings includes: anxiety, guilt, worry, fear, panic, regret, envy, jealousy, and hostility. Together, we could compile a virtually endless list of feelings that many of us know personally. To bring ourselves to energetic health, we would do well to face them all. The way is straightforward: Ask for an image, then correct it.

Rather than suppressing our distressing feelings, some of us may act on them impulsively - one way of retaining a childish attitude to life. This is not an accusation. It is just a description of the development of our lives, the phases that we may not have surmounted in the course of becoming adults.

As we saw earlier, so long as we feel, act, and then think we are not adults, but the slaves of our impulses. The impulses take over and come to dominate us, which leads to a process of diminishment and, perhaps, destructive consequences. We become trapped in our impulses and much of our potential stagnates and atrophies.

But when we use imagery to face our distressing feelings and correct them, we open ourselves to the possibilities within us. We move toward becoming who we are.

Moving Image, Changing Image

How do we know when our imagery is working?

After the angry woman changed the anger into a glass sculpture, she breathed out and opened her eyes. "How do you feel?" I asked. She said: "I feel moved."

The feeling of movement is an important experience in imagery. The image process moves something in us, and *movement equals life*. When we are decaying or in a process of stagnation, we feel a lack of movement – inside, outside, in our lives, physically, emotionally, socially. There is a sense of a loss of movement. And when, through imagery, we feel movement, it means we are restoring ourselves to life. It means the imagery is working and that we are healing.

Sometimes the sense of moving is expressed in changed imagery. For example, one person I worked with had an infected eye. I recommended an exercise where he leaves his apartment and goes to some known healing water that he uses to wash his eye, then retraces the route back to his apartment. He reported to me that the path to the water was a lovely green meadow but that on the way back, the meadow was bursting with flowers. This is a clear sign of movement: two days later, his eye doctor reported that the infected eye was "remarkably" clear.

Re-Applying Our Imagery

I have already explained that if you find you are successful in relieving an ailment through an imagery exercise, you can use the same image whenever the ailment may reappear. This is an important point, because in a number of instances, one application of imagery is not enough to transform distressing feelings.

Even for the woman who created a glass sculpture out of her anger, it would not be surprising if the anger returned in some situations. The relief of a feeling like anger through one transformation does not necessarily mean that the anger has been laid to rest. As I mentioned earlier, feelings are not destroyed, they are mastered. But now, by imaginally creating a glass sculpture out of her anger, the woman has a way of taking charge over it rather quickly, so that the anger no longer overtakes her and creates the conflict and disturbances that it had habitually brought.

Once you have an image that successfully deals with a situation, simply "re-apply" it whenever the need arises.

Troubleshooting

The Other Senses

Some of you may find that when you try to originate your own imagery exercises, the images are vague, perhaps inaccessible. If this happens, then you can focus on another sensory activity, one that you know is strong in you. Instead of saying "see," use the term "hear," or say "touch" or "taste" or "smell." Any of the sensory activities that are available to us can substitute for the visual sense.

Actually, what often happens when you use an alternative sensory activity is that the visual imagery becomes available. But even if this does not happen, if the image remains somehow indistinct, continue your work using the other sensory modalities. This can also include a general sensing called kinesthetic or the movement of musculature called proprioceptive.

There are also several ways to enhance your visual imaging capacity. One practice is to take a book of ordinary landscapes and study a number of them for about 30 to 45 seconds each. Just take a good look at the pictures. Then close your eyes and see if you can see the landscapes one at a time.

A second practice is to recall a scene from your childhood - a place where you used to live, your backyard, the street in front of your building or a room in your home. Just recall it. Then close your eyes and see yourself in that place, the place that you were accustomed to living in for a time.

You can also practice hearing exercises. Hear

sounds that you know – the sound of fish frying in a skillet, glasses clinking in a restaurant, applause in an auditorium. See what happens in your exercises when you do that. Or in the waking state you can smell various spices or perfume essences; or touch different sorts of natural fabrics.

The point is that you can increase your imagery faculty by using familiar scenes, locations or other sensory experiences. Practiced over time, the faculty will begin to grow. You need never be at a loss because you have at least five senses. Play with them and follow those that call forth your imaginings most vividly. See how one sense may help enhance another.

Lighting the Darkness

In your experiences with imagery, you may come to dark places and spaces where you feel afraid - a very common occurrence. It is so common it has a name: "the call into the dark." And there is a very simple technique to handle it.

A woman with whom I worked had cancer. When I asked her to see what the cancer looked like, she saw two monsters in a cave. I asked her if she would be willing to confront the monsters, bringing with her whatever she needed to protect herself. She said she was willing to do that because this was a serious situation for her. So she went to the cave in full battle fatigues with weapons at her command, and as she started to enter the cave, she saw that it was completely dark.

I told her to bring a light with her. Since this was imagination, she could use any light that she wished to dispel the dark so that she could proceed into the cave and confront the monsters directly. She brought a huge searchlight and beamed it into the cave, which enabled her to see more clearly into this dark realm. Now she was willing to enter into the cave to confront the monsters and conquer them.

When we light up the dark we feel safer and are much more willing to enter, explore and confront the monsters within. Sometimes when light penetrates the dark, the demons disappear.

It is very simple to enter into the dark - the place of the unknown, the unfamiliar, the mysterious: You simply take a light with you. In the realm of imagination, you may bring anything you want with you to see your way into the dark.

Similarly, if you feel in any way unsafe, bring any protection that you need - anything you want to wear or use to protect yourself.

The Perfect Rightness of Imagery

One last point, which you no doubt already know.

In doing your imagery work, do not judge yourself or proceed on the basis that there is a right and wrong way to do it or that there is one correct image. If you take this bureaucratic approach, you will defeat yourself. You will become discouraged and want to distance yourself from imagery. There is no right and wrong here, no image that is *the* correct one, no image that is wrong. Forget about all of these ideas. Just do the work. Be interested in the process, not in the product. You will see that almost everyone has the capacity to bring forth spontaneous images or to discover an image. To paraphrase a movie of a few years ago, *Field of Dreams*, "Do it and they will come."

Given all the above, you will discover a new path to health, a new path to life, and perhaps a new path of Spirit, yours to receive through the practical application of this Kabbalah of Light.

Index of Imagery Exercises

About the Author

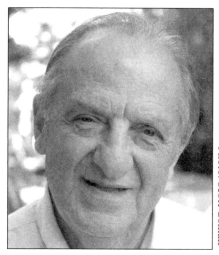

Photo: Scott Osman

Gerald Epstein, M.D., is one of the foremost practitioners of integrative medicine for healing and transformation. He founded and directs the American Institute for Mental Imagery (AIMI), a postgraduate training program for health professionals and an educational center for the public. Dr. Epstein is Assistant Clinical Professor of Psychiatry at Mt. Sinai Medical Center (New York City) and has taught at Columbia University's College of Physicians and Surgeons. Initiated into Visionary Kabbalah by his teacher Colette Aboulker-Muscat, he is a leading exponent and teacher of the Western spiritual tradition and its application to healing and therapeutics.

Dr. Epstein has authored five books and recorded two audios. He maintains a private practice in integrative medicine in New York City where he works with individuals, groups and children. To contact Dr. Epstein, AIMI, or learn more about Visionary Kabbalah call 212-369-4080 or visit: www.drjerryepstein.org.